CALM AND CONFIDENT PARENTING

CALM and CONFIDENT PARENTING

How to Care for Yourself (and Your Kids) through Life's Chaos

Alison Mitzner, MD

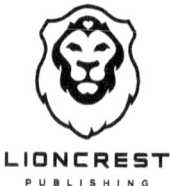

The information in this book is solely for educational purposes and is solely the opinion of Dr. Alison Mitzner, which may differ from other medical professionals. The book does not provide medical advice. The information provided in this book is neither intended nor is implied to be a substitute for professional medical advice. Always seek the advice of your physician about any questions you may have regarding a medical condition or the health and welfare of your child. Never disregard professional medical advice or delay in seeking it because of something you have read in this book.

COPYRIGHT © 2021 ALISON MITZNER, MD

All rights reserved.

CALM AND CONFIDENT PARENTING

How to Care for Yourself (and Your Kids) through Life's Chaos

ISBN   978-1-5445-2194-7   *Hardcover*
          978-1-5445-2193-0   *Paperback*
          978-1-5445-2195-4   *Ebook*

TO MY KIDS, WHO INSPIRE ME EVERY DAY.

CONTENTS

INTRODUCTION 9

1. CALM AND CONFIDENT 19
2. SELF-CARE FOR MOMS 39
3. EMOTIONAL HEALTH 51
4. SLEEP WELL 69
5. EAT WELL 85
6. KEEP MOVING 109
7. TIME MANAGEMENT, ORGANIZATION, AND ROUTINE .. 123
8. CALM AND CONFIDENT PARENTING IN A CRISIS 143

CONCLUSION 159

ACKNOWLEDGMENTS 165

ABOUT THE AUTHOR 167

INTRODUCTION

The countdown to the bus had already begun. How much time was left to get out the door? Fifteen minutes? Ten? Five? Meanwhile, my daughter was in an absolute meltdown over getting dressed. I don't know what exact dress code she thought was in place for that day of school, but the outfit laid out in her room, the one she picked out the night before—the clean, weather-appropriate one—was *not it*. There was a lot of yelling and crying, and not a lot of clothes-wearing.

We were all ready, at baseline, in more than the usual amount of chaos. I was still pretty new at the single mom thing, and we had recently moved into a new apartment. We were all adjusting. And on that day in particular, we were in that transition period, after the kids return to my place, where everything was just a bit extra.

Just as I was trying to simultaneously extricate myself from my daughter's room and will suitable clothes onto her body, my younger one, my son, came in the room grinning and asking me to come to see his "snowfield." The (empty) box of crackers he was toting perhaps should have given me a clue, but I was completely unprepared for what awaited in the living room.

The white-ish coating on the furniture and floors and windowsills did, in fact, create the aforementioned snowfield effect. Or, through grown-up eyes: there were crunched-up crackers sprinkled absolutely everywhere.

"What on earth did you **do**?!?"

I am not sure I managed a great *tone* here, but I'm proud to say that at least my daughter was still the only one yelling and crying.

"I wanted to see what it would look like!" my son happily exclaimed. "I thought it might look like winter."

It was not yet 8:30 a.m.

There are days like this. Every mom knows them. I don't care how much you had life figured out before; everything changes once you have children.

You are just so busy. And stressed. You have no time to sleep. Some days no time to even shower. How are you going to keep everyone happy when you feel like you're running on empty? When are you going to get through a whole day without yelling at the kids?

Never mind getting everything done—how do you even know what to do? How do you know you are doing it right? And how do you take care of everything kid-related without neglecting yourself or your relationships with other adults?

So many moms are overwhelmed, stressed out, and sleep-deprived, often appearing as moody, irritable, and impatient—on top of "mom brain" and plenty of mom guilt. That's before factoring in poor eating and exercise habits, no matter how fit you were in the "before" times.

There's no time to yourself. You feel somehow not up to the job. You might begin to second-guess your parenting decisions or shift from following one source of advice to another and another, depending on who you talked to last.

I've been there…those times when you sit back and close your eyes for a minute and think, *OMG, how in the world am I supposed to manage all this? Can I possibly keep it together? What am I even doing?*

The times when *some*one is having a tantrum because there is no more of the milk they like for breakfast and they have to use *the one in the wrong color carton.*

Those times when you go to the grocery store for milk for breakfast cereal and bread for school lunch and arrive home with bags and bags of groceries…but no milk. (At least you got the bread!)

Those mornings when you know you won't make it to the bus stop on time and there's no time to get the kids to school yourself because you've got a work meeting starting at 8 a.m…and *that's* when your kid announces she peed in the corner instead of the potty.

Then of course, everyday "emergencies" like these are layered over top of the regular assortment of life issues, failing relationships, untenable work demands, and challenging health issues. The croup and the learning disabilities and doctor's warnings about obesity. I've been to all those places too and didn't always feel 100 percent sure I was up to the task.

And I'm a pediatrician as well as a mom, so at least I've got the medical knowledge about how to keep a child healthy and growing on my side. If things can get overwhelming for me, I can see how much more intense it could be for other moms.

Just imagine, though, what it would be like to parent feeling calm and confident. Even when things are chaotic. *Especially* then.

It is possible.

I know because I've been there too.

The truth is, motherhood is many things. It is the best job ever and incredibly rewarding. One thing it is not, though, is easy. Finding things that can make it easier is important for anyone who wants to minimize that pulling-my-hair-out feeling. That's what this book is all about—whatever makes mom life easier, less overwhelming, and more joyful.

I'm here to give my best (science-backed) tips and tricks, drawn from my life as a mom and my expertise as a pediatrician. That expertise makes me a magnet for questions from parents about everything, spanning from: *Do I need to call the doctor?* to *What should I serve for dinner?* or *What can I do about whining?* I can't promise you stress-free parenting—you don't even really *want* everything to be stressless all the time—but I can promise you that you can handle even the most challenging moments of parenting with aplomb. (Or what looks like it, anyway.) I want you to make the most of your time, leave mom guilt behind you, and enjoy mom life to the fullest.

I want you to know—*really know*—that you can handle this.

So much about being a mom is learning as you go. You *don't* always know exactly what you are doing, but you learn from experience. That's especially true of the most difficult experiences. I've had plenty to learn from! A challenging pregnancy, a series of injuries and surgeries, and a difficult marriage and divorce have taught me so much that I would never have known otherwise. All of this has made such a huge impact on who I am as a person—my emotional state, my physical well-being, and how I manage as a busy mom—and, therefore, has had a huge impact on my kids and the people they are growing into.

I'm sharing what I've learned in the hope that it'll give you a shortcut to being a calm and confident parent. I wouldn't want anyone to have to go through what I've been through to learn the things I've learned. To keep yourself and your family healthy and happy. To experience wellness and find balance, even when life is nuts.

To take care of yourself as a way of taking care of your kids—even when one is hollering about the wrong socks, the other is covered in cracker dust, and you're not even out of your pajamas yet.

Standing in the middle of the "snowfield," for a moment

I felt like I would lose it. *The time crunch! The noise! The incredible mess!*

But then, wiser me spoke up. *Okay, I need to take a breath. No one's hurt. She's okay. He's definitely okay. I'm even okay.* In my mind, I quickly ticked through all I'd learned over the years, breathed deeply before doing anything else, and then just kind of clicked into the humorous part of the situation. I looked at my son, and we started laughing and laughing.

I still had too much to do and not enough time to do it, but really, what's better than a kid convinced he can make it snow inside? This is one of the deep joys of parenting, accessing some of what's going on in their awesome little minds as they discover the world.

If I had gone ballistic, what would it even have helped? I'd still have needed to haul out the vacuum, my daughter's clothes would still be wrong, and we'd still be late for the bus. But I also would have missed a "moment" that became a great family memory. And I would have shaped my kids' reactions, too—not for the calmer, that's for sure.

I wrote this book so you, too, can laugh rather than snap when things are definitely *not* going according to plan. (And when is family life ever consistently going according to plan?) You can find calm in the chaos and confidently choose your path.

I'm a single mom of two school-aged kids. I've been in private practice as a pediatrician and served as an attending pediatrician at several of New York City's best teaching hospitals. I've since moved on to a position in the pharmaceutical industry. I have faced my own medical and personal issues, and so it really hit home for me how, even with all my professional knowledge, I didn't feel completely prepared for…*this*. I loved motherhood, but I was undeniably stretched by it, more than I ever imagined I could be.

How in the world do parents ever manage?

My hope is that one of the answers to that question is with this book. It is designed to help moms parent in a way that keeps them and their children feeling calm and confident.

This is not a book to tell you the one right way to parent. There is no one right way! It's also not a book to let you know what you are doing wrong. You are not supposed to know exactly what to do at all times!

In fact, it may surprise you how much of the information in this book isn't really *parenting* information; it's more like wellness information—specifically for moms.

That's the unexpected secret at the core of calm and confident parenting: how you "do" it is by taking good care of yourself. By eating right, getting good sleep (it can be done!), finding time for fitness, practicing self-care, practicing emotional-health hygiene, and discovering ways to manage your stress. Then these healthy habits will "trickle down" to your kids as well.

Even more important, though, is the support these tools provide to you, the mom. They give you the solid foundation you need to proceed with calm and confidence through any kind of parenting day—snowfields included.

1

CALM AND CONFIDENT

There's a reason I named my daughter Serina (meaning peaceful and serene). It says something about my life at the time and my aspirations for myself and my family, as so many names do. She is such a calm child in general, but she does not always embody her name. The morning of The Incorrect Outfit made that clear.

My son actually saved the day that morning—though, I do hope next time he'll find a less crumb-intensive way to do it. The announcement of his experiment shifted the focus off the drama I admit I had been a bit sucked into. I'd been engaging with my daughter's impossible demands for unspecified perfection, and I was frustrated, irritated, and becoming quite impatient.

We can see how well that was working.

After the break my son provided, I was able to step back, take a breath, and return to my daughter calmly, despite the real problems the conflict had created. With confidence behind my renewed efforts, my mood improved and became "contagious" to my daughter, who was able to pull herself together too. And who, as far as I know, did in fact wear clothes to school that day.

The details are a little fuzzy, as I had to immediately shift from laughing with my son back into problem-solving how to get the kids to school (without the bus) and me to my meeting (without my kids). I was only able to do it because I had found that calm place first. When my approach changed, the outcome changed as well.

Had I lost my temper, my daughter might *still* be standing there in a pile of rejected clothes with me carping at her. When it comes to doing my job as a mom, I've never been let down by choosing calm over an angered response.

The most peaceful way to parent is also the most effective. It's about remaining calm and confident, present and patient even when life gets chaotic and you are being pulled in a million directions. It's not necessarily easy, but it is always possible, for any parent. It's a *learned* skill, and, like any other, it requires practice to master. But the tools are here—you can pick them up and use them any time you want.

Parenting is amazing, rewarding…and hard work. And, as we know, sometimes stressful. This is exactly why you want to hone the ability to do it from a calm and confident place. The benefits rebound to you, to your family as a whole, and to your kids (in ways that will influence their entire lives far into the future). It will make your whole life more peaceful and make you a better, happier, healthier parent who is ready to fully enjoy all the moments of mom life.

Here's what makes calm and confident parenting so powerful: kids react differently to a calm parent. When a parent is anxious (not calm), others around them will be anxious. The parent sets the tone, for better or worse. I was recently listening to my son's worries about the next day's visit to his pediatrician. I offered reassurance and empathized with his concerns without contributing whatever stress I had (seeing my kid stressed…). By the end of our brief conversation, my son said, *You always make scary things like the doctor and dentist better, and even fun.* Which I took as a parenting win. Engaging with your children calmly and confidently ensures that, at the very least, you will not add more stress to the mix.

This, of course, is true of interacting with anyone—not just your children. When you are calm, the person you are talking to will feel calmer. (And if you are keyed up, the person you are talking to will feel more keyed up, too.) I've learned this lesson so many times from patients' parents, who tell me, *I feel so much better after talking with you.* I believe I've always given solid advice, but I know a big part of what I have to offer is calm delivery. Parents are often reaching out to me when they are in a stressful place, and one key way I can help is by holding space for calmness.

There's a big-picture angle on calm and confident parenting as well: your kids are watching you, closely observing all your actions and behaviors from the very earliest ages. They learn from you and your example about…everything, really, and that includes how to handle stressful situations. These are lessons that will stay with them into adulthood. What do you want to model for them?

IT ALL STARTS WITH YOU

Calm and confident parenting always begins with you. This means caring for yourself first, before anything or anyone else, because what you do for yourself impacts your entire family. Think about how you parent when you are anxious, stressed, overtired—studies show the operative word in those circumstances will be "impatient"—vs. how you interact when you have optimized your own well-being.

What exactly works varies somewhat from person to person, so you'll have to experiment a bit to find the best strategies for you. A lot of people like to do interior work, like meditation, mindfulness, and yoga. For some, it's more specifically about stress relief, like guided imagery, regular exercise, or even acupuncture.

Upcoming chapters get into detail about many key ways to cultivate calm and confidence through caring for yourself to the same high level of quality as you care for your kids. The central idea is to start with taking best care of mom, so she'll be able to best care for her kids.

In addition to a repertoire of long-term practices that support you in maintaining calm, you'll also want to have in-the-moment strategies on tap for when you need to find a moment of calm within a specific stressful situation. I nominate "take a breath" and "take a break" for most likely to succeed. There's also finding the humor in a situation (as appropriate—like, say, during a living room snowstorm), telling yourself, *This will seem funny*, or calling to mind a favorite mantra/reminder (*Everyone's doing the best they can*, or, *We've been through tough things before*).

MEDITATION

> We have thousands of thoughts per day, and this never ceases to amaze me. Meditation slows our stream of thoughts and helps our minds become more calm, peaceful, and focused. This is a great gift in this nonstop world we live in, when so many of us so easily feel overworked or overwhelmed. Even ten minutes can break through the clutter to find a calmer place.

GET SMART

Knowing that you know what to do in common situations will help you stay calm. The more you know, the more you'll be able to keep calm and carry on. My knowledge of medicine, for example, has kept me even-keeled through many scary parenting moments. (Like, knowing how high a temperature can go before you need to call the doctor.) But you don't have to be an actual expert in anything but yourself, your kids, and your life to rely on your own knowledge base. It's also useful to know what you don't know—and to be open to asking experts to fill in where you have gaps.

GRATITUDE

Research shows that intentionally focusing on feelings of thankfulness is good for you both mentally and physically and can improve your health and the quality of your life in many ways. I'm writing about it here because practicing gratitude makes you more likely to be generous and empathetic toward others, more optimistic, and better able to cope with stress. I'm only extrapolating the teeniest bit here, but I think it's safe to say that gratitude makes you calmer and more confident. So take a moment, every day, to reflect on what is right in your life, and some of the many things you have to be grateful for. Some days it might be harder to dig them out of the morass than others. But they are there. And committing to noticing them can be a life-changer.

FOR THE CHILDREN

OK, so, you *are* also going to take care of your kids. Because of course you are! And you are going to do it best from the place of calm and confidence that you are learning to own.

There are a number of basic things every child needs in place to feel secure, calm, and confident, so we'll start there. Aim to:

- Provide a home that is as safe, familiar, and dependable as possible.
- Encourage your child to express their feelings and ask questions.
- Listen to your child.
- Allow your child opportunities (within reason) to make choices and have control.
- Give plenty of notice if anything is going to change (e.g., family life, job, home, school).

With these operating in the background, children are well prepared to deal when stresses or anxieties arise.

When it does come to an actual stressful situation:

- Be patient with your child.
- Provide information about the situation at hand.
- Validate their feelings.
- Provide reassurance about your child's capabilities.

> **TRADITION!**
>
> Kids love a good tradition, so hold fast to the ones you have. Or start new ones. Or restart traditions from your childhood. This can be as simple as Friday night is pizza night and we rotate who makes a crazy salad. Or as complex as an annual family trip to Florida for winter break. Traditions are great for family bonding and place predictable things on the calendar that the kids can be excited about. There are worse places to lay a foundation for calm and confidence than on "some (fun) things never change".

If your child continues to struggle with stress or anxieties, talk to your pediatrician—they can work with you to find any additional resources you may need.

QUALITY TIME

A main source of mom worry undermining calm and confidence is that you are working too much or aren't around enough for your kids. It is true kids need time with loving, involved, and committed parents, but studies have shown it is quality time that has the biggest positive effect on your children. Kids need "quantity" time too, but what matters more is what is happening during the time you do have. In fact, a smaller amount of quality time is more beneficial than a large quantity of time that's meaningless.

This is why ensuring quality time with your children is one of the best secrets to calm and confident parenting. It makes you feel better; it makes them feel better. They know they are loved and valued; you know you can let go of the guilt and enjoy the relationship.

There is no specific activity that makes time together "quality time." To be valuable and important, quality time requires only that you are truly being with your kids, fully present, and focused on them—no distractions, no other priorities. Protecting this time means ensuring it is uninterrupted and happens regularly. There is no multitasking in quality time. Quality time is interactive time. It is creative time. It is time for communicating and connecting.

Beyond that, do whatever it is your children love to do. It can be as simple as reading books or putting together a puzzle, or some other quiet activity at home. My children light up when I sit on the floor with them and play whatever game they choose (or make up) or listen to them read to me now that they are able to turn the tables that way. Cooking is great. Crafts are great. Athletic games are great. Unstructured play is great. Anything outside is even better.

Playing with your children, no matter what you actually do, is so valuable—even if it lasts just fifteen or twenty minutes. There are so many benefits for your children when you play with them, but the biggest one for you is that it's an opportunity to be fully engaged with them in their world. Doing things that are fun and calming with your kid—the parent sets the tone—creates increased connection, which results in children feeling more secure, more confident, and less stressed.

Even when it's raucous fun, quality time with your kids is a little oasis in your day, regardless of whatever else is going on, and that's renewing for all of you.

There were times when my children were younger that I was "playing" with them but in my head I was thinking of all I had to do and feeling all that stress instead of enjoying the game. Eventually I realized what I was doing and decided to take my own advice instead.

The secret to getting my head in the game was using organizational strategies, along the lines of what you'll read about in Chapter 7. This included some protected time with my kids, as well as designated times for all the other "stuff" I had to do, so I could enjoy being with my kids, secure in the knowledge the other things were done, or soon would be. (And that I wouldn't forget them if I stopped running over them in my mind!)

I'm not saying you will never need or want the TV to be a babysitter. Of course, now and then you will still need time to get chores done or take that work call at home. Not to mention, you want your children to be able to play independently and know how to be creative themselves. You cannot plan every moment of every day to be filled with Very Meaningful Interactions with your kids, because you live in the real world.

But kids remember the wonderful quality times that you do create—they're as likely to hold onto the memory of that one song you always sang at the top of your lungs together on long car rides as they are the huge vacation spectacular you planned for months. Making quality time together a priority sends a clear message to kids about how important they are to you and how much you love and care for them.

It's a feeling they'll still have on the nights you have to work late, or the times you travel for work, or the days somehow taken up entirely by errands.

UNSTRUCTURED PLAY

Many moms feel most comfortable with structured activities with their kids, but unstructured play is absolutely crucial for child development. Whether or not it is part of your quality time with your child, make time and space for your child to engage in unstructured play every day. Let kids be kids. (Bonus points for anything outdoors.)

One major study showed children who have regular unstructured outside play time are smarter, more social, less aggressive, healthier, and happier. Unstructured play is important for motor skills practice, hands-on exploring, social interaction, problem-solving, focus, emotional well-being, and creativity. The American Academy of Pediatrics recommends free play daily, citing the importance to children's physical and mental health, as well as their social learning. Aim for at least an hour a day.

Most importantly, spending quality time with your children will help them when they are feeling stressed. The same goes for you: having that quality time every day (OK, most days) will help keep you in the calm and confident zone as well.

This quickly becomes a virtuous circle: when you are focused, well rested, and calm, think about how you are able to interact with your child compared with when you are stressed, sleep-deprived, anxious, multitasking, and dealing with every other thing on your mind except your kid. The calmer and more confident your daily interactions, the more quality time will be available—time that you're *not* spending in conflict over who can't find their shoes or whatnot—and the more present you'll be to that time. And the more you'll enjoy quality time and make the most of it, the more it will bolster you in your pursuit of calm and confidence.

TO CONNECT, DISCONNECT

"Mom, I like your No Screen Time After Dinner rule."

—MY SON, AFFIRMING THE DECREE I ACTUALLY LIKE TO THINK OF AS THE QUALITY TIME AFTER DINNER RULE.

This one is crucial: The first rule of quality time is that nobody is on the phone for quality time. Connection time is digital disconnection time.

SCIENCE IS NOT KIND TO PARENTS ON PHONES

The research around the effects on children of their parents' use of devices is downright alarming. Studies show that kids act out more when they are competing with an electronic device for their parents' attention. And, sadly, the kids are right: they may well be losing that competition. Some parents literally don't see or hear their kids while their focus is on their phone or other device, and are irritable when interrupted while on their phones.

To kids, all our staring at our phones, answering every "ping" on the spot, looks like they aren't interesting to us, or they are boring or don't matter to us. The research reveals kids get angry at the devices, and experts say the emotional consequences go far beyond frustration in the moment. The bottom line: Look up. Are your kids there? Put. Down. Your. Phone.

If you are on your phone or other device, you are not having quality time. Don't check email, don't open Instagram, don't read texts, and don't browse the web "for just a minute." When you are with your kids, be with your kids. Be 100 percent focused on them.

For something that is so often in short supply, it is a crime not to take full advantage of your time when you do have it. When everyone involved disconnects, you'll all be able to enjoy the quality time, however much of it you are able to grab.

I recommend working together with your children to set aside specific times for the whole family to disconnect. This is how my family came to our strict policy against screens between dinner and bedtime—and how my kids bought in. If you were wondering how much real quality time with their parents means to kids, they'll happily give up yet another video game for it. But only if you are really there for it, and them.

Make a plan for limiting tech time that works for your family—starting with family meals as designated no-tech times, to ensure regular uninterrupted face-to-face connections with the most important people in your life. I also recommend a no-tech zone before bedtime, for everyone. If your kids know you do it too, they'll be more likely to comply.

THE UPS AND DOWNS OF DISCONNECTING

Having protected time disconnected from technology is good not only for your family and your own sanity but also for your child—in a whole host of ways beyond appreciating family time. Decreasing tech time has a long-lasting positive impact on educational achievement, social skills, and face-to-face interpersonal relationships.

The downsides of out-of-control tech time are equally impactful. Large amounts of time spent with screens are associated with decreased playtime, physical activity, hands-on learning, sleep, and, yes, family time—all key points of learning for children.

FAMILY DINNERS

This is always a favorite way to get in quality time, but one that is too often hard to arrange into our busy schedule. My advice is: do what you can to find a way to make it work for your family. It will be worth it. According to The Family Dinner Project, spearheaded by two women at Harvard, research over the past twenty years has shown that "sharing a fun family meal is good for the spirit, brain, and health of all family members."

Family dinner is not about the meal itself. It is about the family gathering to enjoy it together and reconnect over it. Spending this time with your children at the dinner table really makes the family feel bonded. Kids get that sense of belonging, which research shows increases their self-esteem. Bonus: you will get a window into what is going on with your children. Also, the family that eats together is calmer together.

Just like for any quality time, there is one rule for family dinners: no phones at the table. For adults or kids. No TV, either.

From there, whatever else you do around the table should be what fits your family, and it will probably shift and change over time.

Try to keep the talk around the table light and fun. Save the "serious" talks for another time. Ask your children about their day, but do more than just say, "How was your day?" Ask direct and specific questions to open the door for more than just a "good," "fine," "okay" answer.

For example, ask, "What was the topic in math class today?" or "What did you do in gym?" Ask what made them laugh today. Ask them about what they may have read. You can also discuss their favorite activities, hobbies, pets, family outings—whatever engages them if they are not interested in discussing their day. There are many online sources for suggested topics at the dinner table and even decks of cards with questions to prompt discussion. This kind of conversation helps them know you are interested in them and proud of them, and they will open up more in response.

Family dinner does not have to be every night. It doesn't even have to be dinner. Lots of families have special routines around weekend breakfasts or Sunday lunch. Do whatever appeals to you, but know that more is better. Once a week is better than once a year. The benefits of family dinner should be in balance with all the other demands on your time. If it is making everyone nuts to fit in that third night a week, that might not be the right rhythm for your family, at least not right now. So start small and be realistic.

You may also want to involve your kids in planning and making these dinners. Having a shared project with a desirable outcome—*I want the spaghetti and meatballs we learned to make from Grandpa!*—is great quality time. In addition, studies show kids who regularly participate in these ways make healthier food choices as adults.

Set a time (though don't expect the meal to always land on the table at that exact time), and stick to it. That way, everyone knows what to expect, and you're more likely to follow through. Your kids will probably hold you to it too!

Life happens. After-school activities may change so Tuesdays don't work anymore. A doctor's appointment may interfere, or someone may feel sick, so you'll have to miss or reschedule a day. Over time, you may be able to add family dinner days or subtract them. What matters is the priority you place on time together.

THE JOY OF MUSIC

One of my family's favorite ways to enjoy quality time together is to make it musical. The best part about music, for us, is that it's fun. I've always loved music—making it, listening to it, dancing to it—and have made it a big part of my life. Enjoying music together is a big part of what makes it such a good bonding event to make, listen, or dance to music together.

Music also comes with a whole load of powerful benefits, and that is especially true in the realm of de-stressing and creating calm. I don't really have to tell you this, though: most of us just know we feel better with music. It can help us relax, reduce our stress, motivate us when we're tackling challenges, and help us fall asleep and sleep deeper at night. Music improves our well-being and helps us become more mindful and present.

You don't have to be a good singer or smooth dancer or know how to play an instrument to reap the benefits of music being a regular part of your family life. Doing any of those things poorly will do the trick, as long as you are enjoying it. You could never play or sing or dance and still reap the benefits from simply listening to music.

Like anything else, you don't want to push something on your children that they are not interested in. But when you're following your child's interest, music, in whatever form, is great.

My kids and I love nothing better than to sing along to a favorite song, breaking out silly dance moves. Sometimes I'll play the piano for our singalongs (or try to play guitar, which I'm still learning). Sometimes music helps us wind down, and sometimes it revs us up. But it always adds smiles, and laughter, and calm to our day. Whatever the mood, music is always part of quality time for us.

WHY MUSIC LESSONS RULE

If your children have an interest in learning to play a musical instrument, I highly recommend it. The process comes with so many benefits, including improving academic performance, enhancing social and physical skills, and increasing discipline and patience. Playing an instrument helps develop self-motivation and persistence and increases confidence.

You don't really need any more reasons to root for your child to take up an instrument. But let me just point out how many of the benefits feed directly into creating calm and confidence in your child—and thereby your home. So this is an effort that's so worth it—even before you factor in what a gift it is to learn something they can enjoy throughout their entire lives!

CALM MOM

Learning to stay calm amid chaos has been a complete game-changer for me, long after my daughter decided to just get her own self dressed every morning and my son caved to the reality of outside-only snow. It's made me a better, happier parent all around to make the changes I needed in my own life—starting with the self-care we'll discuss in the next chapter—to give me that ability to find calm.

Also key: learning the small but important changes to make in my kids' lives for the same reason. It's all allowed me to be more patient and present as a mom. My kids are surely happier as well—aside from moods being contagious, who wouldn't prefer a calm mom over the alternative?

Of course, life is still chaotic. There's always going to be stress—and it's okay to feel stressed. It's how you handle it that matters. Calm and confident parenting doesn't mean you are always automatically calm. It does mean you know how to get there when you need to. It means you know it's possible, even in the midst of chaos.

2

SELF-CARE FOR MOMS

Wednesday night is my singing night. I sing with a group of women who get together for a couple of hours to sing everything from pop songs to some more meditative, mindful stuff, accompanied by guitar or piano. It's also a group of moms socializing, catching up, empathizing, and generally remembering how free time with adults works. Once in a while, the group meets up at someone's house for dinner or performs at the Y or at different events and venues.

For a long time, this group was an important part of my mom self-care—something I loved to do, something I was doing just for me, something social. After work on Wednesdays, I'd be tired, work-stressed, and wondering if I was right to ask the sitter to stay late. *Ugh, should I really go? Maybe an early night at home instead…*

What always got me there was knowing how much better I felt seeing this group of friends. When I'd get there, all the other moms were basically in the same boat. Chatting, connecting, and *singing* always makes me happy. (In fact, we know from studies singing improves our mood and decreases stress by releasing endorphins, producing serotonin, and decreasing cortisol.) Singing with others, that's even better. We'd all come in just beat from whatever was going on in our days and end up staying late because we were having so much fun.

YOU FIRST

Moms are all about their kids, putting them first. Unfortunately, but understandably, this sometimes means putting themselves and their needs on the back burner. Ultimately, though, this does more harm than good. The most important thing you can do as a mom is to take good care of yourself. That *is* how you take care of your kid. Everything you do to increase your well-being will support you in being a better parent and improve your children's well-being as well. Science says it is so: taking time for yourself makes you more likely to enjoy mom life, and that creates clear, positive effects on your children.

Self-care is where it all starts. It's important for your overall health and well-being—physical, mental, and emotional. It improves your mood, makes you less stressed and anxious, and makes you happier, more focused, more productive and energetic, and better able to parent. It's how you stay present, patient, and calm. Self-care is not selfish—it's how you make your best self available to others. It's how you make the most of mom life.

WHAT IS SELF-CARE?

Self-care is anything we do to improve our own health, well-being, and happiness. It's doing something for *you*. It's prioritizing things you enjoy or perhaps don't so much enjoy but know will benefit your health and happiness in the long run. It doesn't just mean manicures and spa days, or anything fancy or splurge-y. It can also mean getting to that annual checkup, fitting in a workout somehow, or decluttering that closet that irks you every time you open it.

The remaining chapters in this book are, essentially, different forms of self-care. Getting good sleep, eating well, working out (my go-to self-care when I'm feeling overwhelmed), prioritizing emotional health, getting organized, managing your time, and prepping for emergencies—these are all ways to improve your well-being. It's the same as the groundwork for feeling calm and confident as a mom.

Those chapters obviously tend toward the practical, but they are not a comprehensive list of ways to perform self-care. Self-care will look a little different for everyone.

You'll know best what works for you. There are a few factors everyone should look out for:

- Time to yourself.
- Time to focus on your interests and do something you love. Not all self-care is intrinsically enjoyable, but the *best* self-care is.
- Time with friends and, generally, the people who mean the most to you (aside from your kids). We know that social connections improve our physical, mental, and emotional well-being, increasing happiness and lowering anxiety. And as parents, we role model to our kids the importance of enjoying, and nurturing, friendships and family relationships.
- Time to de-stress.
- Time in community.

Notice a theme? If not for this, then what are time management skills even for? Self-care is not just going to magically happen if you don't find the time and protect it.

Look for small things you can fit into any day just because they make you happy or healthy. I've got a friend who insists on grinding her own beans for the first cup of coffee for the day, just to get that smell. Another puts a new song on her playlist each day.

Schedule in real time for self-care too, even if it's just fifteen minutes at a time. Take more when you can get it, but, most of the time, an hour or less is all you *need* to benefit. A drink with a friend, a cat nap, a walk outside, a quick meditation…what you choose is just personal preference. What matters is that you choose something meaningful to you.

UNPLUG

In the same way unplugging brings benefits to your children and to family time, disconnecting gives you benefits too, allowing you to really recharge your mind and body. Not saying you have to go cold turkey or give up technology, but reserving some pieces of your life away from devices brings immediate and lasting improvements in your quality of life, increasing your health, and happiness, your mental clarity, concentration and creativity, even your fitness level.

Consider designating certain times and spaces to be tech no-go zones *for you*. No tech at family meals, no tech before you get out of bed in the morning, and definitely no tech during self-care activities! (OK, I'll allow phones for *emergency* contact, and a quick photo or two.)

When you disconnect, you'll find more time in your day—time you could use for quality time or self-care. A University of Maryland study looked at "a day without media" and showed that those who unplugged reported more time with friends and family, more time exercising, and even healthier food choices.

BE KIND TO YOURSELF

This kind of self-care is more challenging to many moms: go easy on yourself. Give yourself a little grace. There is no perfect parent, and that's okay. You know you are doing your best. Think of it this way: your kids are always going to think you're the best (even when they say the opposite sometimes). Why not believe them?

MOM BRAIN

A great time to practice being kind to yourself is when you've had an episode of mom brain—missed a pickup or a bill or called your kid the dog's name. In my family, The Time Mom Burned the Pasta and Then Dropped the Replacement Pasta on the Floor lives in infamy.

First, know that you are not alone. We've all been there (and lived to tell the tale).

Second, be assured the brain fog is real and physiological—not permanent.

Third, realize that for the most part, people will be understanding.

Finally, don't worry you'll forget the really important stuff. You won't!

...Oh, and fifth! (See? Mom brain.) Self-care is often the best solution, typically coming down to the most obvious: get some sleep.

Here are some ways to be kind to yourself even (or especially) when things get tough.

Learn to say "no." You don't have to do *every*thing. Say yes to the things that make you happy and align with your wants, needs, and goals. But draw the line as needed. Give yourself a break.

Admit that some things are not worth stressing over. It's totally normal and okay to feel sad or anxious or angry when the situation demands it. But not everything demands it. Aim to keep perspective.

Forgive yourself. You're a mom, but you're also a human, and you've got one of the hardest jobs in the world. Sometimes you're going to lose it. Sometimes you are going to raise your voice in anger. Sometimes you are going to be late for the pickup from soccer practice. You are going to make mistakes. It happens. You're trying. Forgive yourself.

Banish mom guilt. That feeling when your child asks if you could stay at home with him all the time. The mom guilt is real, but you can't let yourself fall into the trap of neglecting yourself in an attempt to banish that guilt, like canceling plans with friends for more time with your kids. They're likely to be asleep before you leave or within five minutes after you leave anyway! Remember it's the quality of your time together that actually matters. Giving up things you need to do for work or for self-care is not going to make you feel better anyway, so don't hang onto guilt for it.

Practice gratitude. It only takes a little extra effort and a couple of minutes a day to pause and consider what you are grateful for. I like to do this as a check-in before I go to sleep. It's also a great way to start the day. It still amazes me how much even a brief focus on gratitude can change.

UNSOLICITED ADVICE

Every mom knows you're going to get plenty of advice, whether you want it or not. Seems like everyone has an opinion on how you should or shouldn't do things, and they are in a big hurry to tell you all about it.

My advice about unsolicited advice? For the most part, ignore it. Taking good care of yourself means learning to trust yourself and not letting others' opinions throw you off course.

Tasha, a mom friend of mine, learned all about this early in her experience of motherhood. A few months in, she began making her own baby food, and once she started, she found she really enjoyed puréeing and combining and packing up. The process was somehow relaxing, and she felt good about giving her baby the freshest, healthiest food and knowing exactly what was in everything. There are a lot of things in life and motherhood that can't be controlled, but this little corner of her world could go just how she wanted. For Tasha, this chore was actually a nice little bit of self-care.

And then her girlfriends started weighing in. Turned out, they had a lot of opinions about which foods she should and shouldn't offer, and when and how she should and shouldn't prepare them.

You have to strain it. He could choke.

I read giving him that increases the risk of allergies.

Doesn't he need more protein?

This was stressing Tasha out. She began second-guessing herself, even though she had made this plan with her pediatrician. Was this the best thing for her baby? The well-meaning "input" was also ruining the positive vibe Tasha had been getting from baby food making. And new moms, especially, need all the peaceful, undemanding moments they can get.

I've had plenty of similar experiences as a mom. There are people who take it upon themselves to tell a pediatrician how to deal with kids, so I am sure moms undefended by academic credentials get so much more. Every time it happens, I have to remind myself it's just outside noise. I'm doing fine. My kid is doing fine. This person is entitled to their opinion, and they can follow that opinion with their kid. But I don't need to change what I'm doing just because I heard this advice.

My (solicited) advice to Tasha was not exactly what she wanted to hear in the moment, because no, I didn't have the power to stop the flow of "helpful" information. What I said to her was this:

This is going to happen a million times. Everyone has their opinions, and they are going to share them with moms whether or not they want them or ask for them. So here's what you do: Block it out. Nod. Say, "OK." Then move on. Carry on doing what you were doing, your way. As long as you are comfortable with it, you are good to go. Trust yourself.

Trust but verify. If you are not 100 percent confident in your approach, whatever it is, check in with your pediatrician—an actual expert. Choose one or two people as trusted advisors, and don't worry about what others say. All that unsolicited advice will just overwhelm and stress you.

It's not like you'll never update your ideas. It's just that you don't want to ping from one thing to another because you lack confidence in your parenting decisions. There's no avoiding unsolicited advice. But letting what's not right for you roll off your back is a key skill for calm and confident parenting and a foundational kind of self-care.

SELF-CARE WHEN YOU NEED IT MOST

Self-care is most important when it seems most impossible to fit into your life.

Parenting is hard work, and if you are stressed, overworked, or burned out, you are going to struggle. You'll be more impatient or irritable, definitely less efficient, and you'll miss out on the joy of it all. And isn't accessing that joy the whole point of all the hard work?

So sing with a bunch of other moms, even when you'd swear you were too tired to do so. Or switch off your screens and meet up with a friend to exercise, even if you have to get a sitter. Keep on making the baby food, even if you have to tune out what your favorite aunt has to say about it.

Do whatever it is you need to do to take care of yourself. Improve your well-being to improve your parenting to improve your child's experience of their family and their world.

Do more of what you love to benefit those you love—both your children and yourself.

3

EMOTIONAL HEALTH

Emotional health is a crucial part of overall health for parents as well as children. I'm writing about it here, however, because emotional health is the foundation you need for being able to stay calm in the midst of chaos, including family life chaos. When you are emotionally healthy, you are a better, calmer, more confident parent. And, moreover, an amazing role model for your kids and *their* emotional health.

You can learn to understand, manage, and work with your emotions. As you improve your emotional health, you'll be healthier and happier. You'll be more productive, too, in all aspects of life. You will, overall, feel so much better about yourself and enjoy your family life to the fullest. You'll find it easier to keep whatever comes up in perspective, handling issues with fewer setbacks. You'll feel more in control of your behavior as well as your feelings.

STRESS

No one escapes without stress, and being a parent is often a whole layer of it.

Actually, you don't want to escape stress. Not entirely. Stress can be productive. It is good when we need to react to urgent situations, and it helps us stay motivated. It can help us be more efficient and get more things done.

When it takes over your life, though, becoming intense and/or continuous, that's when stress becomes harmful. Emotionally, it can cause anxiety, worry, and depression, which can worsen sleep, diet, and more. Increased stress also affects the immune system, and those who are more stressed are more susceptible to infection and other health problems.

So what's important is not to avoid stress, but to know how to handle it. Reap the benefits of stress where they exist, but learn to keep stress in check so it does not get to the point of causing unwanted physical symptoms or emotional impacts.

Maintaining emotional health is the bedrock for calm and confident parenting.

Emotional health is just as important as physical health, and, in fact, the two are closely intertwined. Good emotional health leads to better physical health, including lower blood pressure, lower risk of heart disease, and maintaining a healthy weight. How you care for and deal with your physical health also impacts your emotional health.

It is our reactions to our feelings—not the feelings themselves—that can impact our emotional health. The goal is to be able to regulate our emotions and our reactions to handle them in ways that won't stress us out or make things worse.

Does emotional health mean you need to be (or appear) happy all the time? Of course not—no one is. You have moods, capital F "Feelings," and, let's not forget, a good measure of unpredictability in your life that just comes with your "mom" job title. So let's start improving emotional health right now by agreeing not to hold ourselves to impossible standards.

What emotional health does mean is that you are in good control of your emotions—the good, the bad, and the ugly. To be a good emotional regulator, you need to be more aware of your emotions (and your reactions to your emotions) than many people are. And the good news is this is a skill that can be learned.

DO IT YOURSELF

There are plenty of ways to pursue improved emotional health with the assistance of professionals of various kinds, and if that's of interest and available to you, I recommend it. But there are also a few underappreciated options for improving your emotional health you can do on your own.

MINDFULNESS OF EMOTIONS

Emotional health begins to optimize as you increase your awareness of your feelings and your reactions to them. This starts by simply noticing emotions when you have them and tracking the emotions you have. As this becomes habitual, you'll begin to notice, too, how you react to those emotions.

A key part of this process is acceptance of the emotions you have. It is okay to feel sad or mad or afraid—or joyful or loving, for that matter. It's normal! Where we run into trouble is when we nurture unhelpful reactions to those feelings by snapping at someone or trying to suppress the feeling, for example.

The ability to stay on an even keel despite turbulent emotions—to not overreact or take things personally—truly does keep you at peace. To stay strong (calm) on the outside, stay strong (calm) on the inside. It's not always easy, but it is always worth it.

TEACH YOUR CHILDREN WELL

We're going to get into this more later in the chapter, but a parent's job includes inculcating emotional health in their children. You do this in a few ways, but one of them is explicit instruction. And when you are offering your children good advice in this area, listen to yourself! Make sure you are practicing as you preach. If you're offering good counsel, it would be a shame not to take advantage of it in your own life.

SUPPORT SYSTEM

Don't expect to magically maintain good emotional health all by yourself. When it comes to parenting, the key support for a lot of people is a solid Mom Tribe. I've learned the most about daily life parenting from people going through more or less what I'm going through. Sometimes, the best thing you can hear is just, "Me, too." A little bit of been-there, done-that empathy can be very calming. So is just knowing you are not alone, or losing it.

Call on the support systems around you to aid you in your quest. If you don't feel you have adequate support in place, then do the work necessary to build up your network, formal and informal. It's not easy, but that time is always a worthy investment.

Ideally, you want a selection of people from outside your immediate family. You might draw on different people for different things. The shoulder you want to cry on might not be attached to the person you ask to drive you to the ER if you ever need it. What's important is that you can see and feel the cheering squads and safety nets in your world.

You do have to make sure this tribe is a positive tribe. It's possible for mom-to-mom interaction to be guilt-inducing, or full of subtle mom-bashing, or too superficial to represent real mom life—and you're better off with no one than a tribe like that!

SELF-CARE

Self-care is so important to overall well-being, most definitely including emotional health, that it got its own chapter. Remember, the important point is to take care of yourself before you take care of anyone else—even when that *anyone else* is your child. Or you won't be in a position to provide the best care.

EXERCISE

My personal favorite when it comes to managing my emotions is to take advantage of the connections between physical and emotional health, and move. Exercise is a great way to reduce stress and feel energized, even if you get just fifteen or twenty minutes. It clears your mind, sharpens your thinking, builds resilience and mental toughness, and improves coping skills.

When exercise releases endorphins in your brain, it physiologically makes you feel good. It can also just provide a little space when you're working through something—a simple "time out." Exercise promotes feelings of relaxation, calmness, positivity, and improved self-esteem and an overall sense of well-being.

What better way to combat overwhelm of various kinds?

For me, vigorous exercise triggers these emotional advantages. For many people, yoga or something similarly meditative works better for this purpose.

MEDITATION

The benefits of meditation, mindfulness practices, and relaxation techniques for many aspects of your health and wellness are already famous. If they are a good fit for you, they are great tools in regulating emotions, managing stress, and promoting relaxation. They aren't for everyone or may take some practice before you do find them helpful. Guided meditation is a great starting point for anyone new to meditation or those finding it hard to relax their mind on their own, or struggling to stick with a practice. In any case, the bar to entry is low—why not give it a try?

BREATHE

Take a breath. Your mom might have told you, and perhaps you've even said it to your kids, but it remains good advice for everyone, including you. Simply focusing on your breath, and breathing in and out fully and slowly a few times, is calming and can at times be all you need to proceed purposefully rather than reactively.

There are physiological benefits to pausing for a few moments of deep breathing that will put you in a better place emotionally. Breathing is a good way to interrupt and redirect an unhelpful reaction to emotion. It can help you relax a bit, clear your mind, prepare to think about why you are doing what you are doing, and push forward productively. That might or might not mean changing your path, but pausing to breathe will help you prepare for forward motion one way or the other.

ACUPUNCTURE

In the quest to maintain positive emotional health, I say, let's make use of all the tools available to us. When a colleague recommended acupuncture to me ten years ago, I was hesitant to try. I could hardly believe it would do anything. But since I was struggling with an injury myself, I decided I had nothing to lose. I am so grateful I added it to the conventional Western medicine approaches I was also using! Experiencing the benefits firsthand changed my world.

While I first used acupuncture for particular symptoms while I was waiting to get a diagnosis, I want to recommend it now for its ability to reduce stress and improve overall well-being. Like anything else, if you try it and it doesn't turn out to be for you, try something else! (Always be sure to go to a properly trained and licensed acupuncturist.)

JOB ONE

Emotional health is as important for your kids as it is for you. The more solid your children's emotional health is, the easier it is for you to be a calm and confident parent—the same equation as for your own emotional health.

Facilitating your children's emotional health is one of your biggest jobs as a parent. And you are already doing it every day, in many important ways.

FOCUS ON DAY-TO-DAY RELATIONSHIPS

Daily interactions with your children provide an ever-renewing source of opportunities to model emotional health—or to blow it. (Luckily, there's always another chance coming to do better.) Engaging with your children patiently and calmly even—or especially—when things get chaotic is so beneficial.

Your relationship with your child is foundational to their emotional health. The bond itself is powerful. It lays the foundation for their behaviors, choices, and personality—both now and as they develop over time. It impacts their physical, mental, and emotional health. When children are secure in the relationship, they not only grow up happier, but they develop a better ability to regulate their emotions in stressful and difficult situations.

You set the emotional tone for your kids. When you are calm, they will be calmer. When you are anxious, their anxiety will escalate. This is because moods and emotions are contagious. This science-backed fact is never clearer than in the interactions between parents and children.

Role modeling matters as much for emotional health as for all the other things your kids will absorb from you. From their observation of you, they will take lifetime lessons about handling emotion and stress and discussing and expressing feelings. And they pick up on everything!

Let them see how you regulate your emotions, including when you are upset, and how you react to feelings. When they see you calmly reacting in stressful situations, they will learn to stay calm even when they are anxious or faced with a stressful situation.

A calm approach in chaotic times will not only avoid adding more stress, it will also actually have a calming effect on your child and on the situation itself. Additionally, when you are calm, your children will actually hear and be able to absorb more of what you are saying to them, both about what to do in that exact moment and also about what to do (or not do) in general.

LEARN TO COMMUNICATE

Kids feel it whether they are (or aren't) being treated with kindness, respect, and love. No surprise, kids listen more to any message that is delivered in a calm, loving tone than to anything loud or harsh.

How you talk with your children is so important—not just to any given situation, but to your relationship as a whole. The words you choose, your tone, whether or not you are fully present as you speak—it will all influence how successfully you connect, how your child will react within themselves, and how they will respond to you.

Children need to learn to express emotions appropriately. You can help them learn how to do so in a positive way—even when the emotion doesn't feel positive. Whether a child is frustrated, angry, sad, or anything else, normalize the feeling and the power of feelings in general.

Talking about feelings is a crucial skill, and your children learn their most important lessons about it from you. How do they learn? By doing. So don't hide your own feelings or minimize theirs. Let your kids know it is okay to share their feelings. And not just okay, but important!

Validate your child's emotions as they come up. Asking an upset child to stop crying, or to calm down, is asking them to push aside their emotions—and that's the opposite of what they need. Crying is a good thing if they are sad. Getting angry is okay as long as it is expressed productively.

Do not brush your child's feelings aside, including when their upset or stress stems from something that seems like it isn't a big deal. It might still be a huge deal to a child, and they are entitled to their feelings. Don't tell kids they are fine when they are fearful. Reassure them, or provide additional information to decrease their worry, but do not mask or deny the truth of the situation. With practice confronting the reality of their fears, kids can learn to cope when difficult things arise, just as adults do.

When you minimize their feelings, this can make them feel as if their emotions are wrong. You are teaching them they shouldn't be sharing their feelings. You risk them suppressing or not sharing their emotions, and when they do that, they cannot get practice in dealing with feelings in an effective way.

Instead, talk to them about whatever is happening that is

stirring up emotion (positive or negative) to discover what might be causing the stress. Talk over what the emotion feels like and what they can do if they need to manage it. Let them hear you discuss your feelings, too, and how you manage them (remember: role model). Talk with your kids about their worries, listen to what they say, and help them figure out how they can deal with them.

Direct instruction is another key way you help your children learn to handle emotions. They get a lot by osmosis, and those are extremely powerful lessons.

Teach and model:

- That emotions are not a permanent state and will rise and fall with circumstances
- Resilience
- Words for their feelings and the way feelings create physical sensations
- How they can soothe themselves without covering up their emotions
- Empathy, respect, and kindness
- How to apologize and make amends when something has happened within a relationship
- Frustration, mistakes, and failure, and love, accomplishment, and joy

Dealing with emotions is not a skill anyone is born with, so all children need to be taught how to do it. That includes specific, if simple, explanations, directions, and practice.

MANAGE STRESS

Parents may not always recognize stress in a child's life because adults may not perceive the same things as stressful as children do. Plus, kids are resilient and usually adapt to change and challenges fairly well. But there are times when stresses, big or small, can take a toll. If unaddressed, childhood stress can lead to anxiety and may cause physical and mental health issues in the future.

As parents, we need to be able to identify when stress is negatively affecting our children and teach them how to cope with it. Just as with adults, the aim is not to avoid or remove all stress, even if that were possible. Experiencing stress is part of how they learn to identify and cope with it—a skill that will apply all through their lives. However, we can help children avoid and/or manage the stress that is continuous or intense.

Stress affects the body, behavior, and emotions in a variety of ways—some of them unexpected—and it can impact children of any age. Kids are resilient, but stress will take a toll if they are not, in fact, handling it well. Here are some signs and symptoms that let you know your child may need more help dealing with their stress:

- Mood swings
- Acting out
- Changes in sleep or sleep disruptions like nightmares or fear of the dark
- Decrease in appetite or loss of interest in food
- Crankiness or irritability
- Inability to relax
- Unwillingness to participate in school
- Bed-wetting
- Headaches
- Fear of strangers
- Clinginess
- Excessive crying

You know your child better than anyone, so when you notice changes, take seriously the implicit messages those changes carry. If they are not resolved by making a little extra time for your child each day, listening carefully to what they say, and offering plenty of information and reassurance, then it's time to talk to your pediatrician.

DO THESE THREE THINGS EVERY DAY

If you want your children to feel loved while also helping them to be confident and internally motivated, I've got three everyday strategies for you. These encourage your children to be more self-assured, resilient, curious, creative, self-sufficient, and *calm*, and they generally promote strong emotional health. They are:

1. Give them choices and control.
2. Allow them to try to solve their own problems.
3. Provide positive reinforcement.

Choices allow children to feel more in control and therefore give them confidence and greater self-sufficiency. This is everything from having a toddler choose which shirt they want to wear or what fruit they want in their lunch, to having an older child choose which after-school activity to sign up for or which books to read for daily free reading.

Problem-solving on their own does not mean kids never need or want your help. Many times they will directly ask for it. But don't get out in front of everything that comes their way. Give kids the chance to address or resolve things before you get involved, and let them know you have full confidence in their ability to handle them. Provide support, of course, but let your child take the lead. This develops both competence and confidence. They will know you have their back—but that you are not going to do for them what they can do for themselves.

When my kids ask for help with something, I've learned to say, *I'll be right there*, and wait a bit before I go see what's up. A minute later, checking in with them, I usually hear,

I did it, I did it! They are excited about their independent success. Over time, this increases confidence and self-motivation.

Positive reinforcement means highlighting (and thereby promoting) good behavior. Often parents focus on the negative without even really realizing it, but it's more powerful to "catch them being good." This will increase confidence and internal motivation.

Positive reinforcement—sometimes as simple as saying, "Nice work there"—can be added into the day for efforts great and small, whether it is brushing teeth without a reminder, completing a chore without grumbling, inviting a new friend to play, venturing to try a different sport, persisting through a complicated school assignment, or any other challenge.

Be sure to praise them when they solve their own problems or try something new or difficult—regardless of the outcome. Always praise the effort along the way and, if and when they don't get to their desired result, give encouragement for the attempt. Point out any problem-solving, flexibility, learning, and growth. This kind of acknowledgment and encouragement makes them feel excited and competent.

These are all campaigns you can begin when your child is

very young, and though they will begin to look different over time, they will remain useful as your child matures.

How you care for yourself and how you parent are key to developing and maintaining emotional health for the entire family. You have a big role in creating and supporting your children's emotional health.

Fortunately, you also have an automatic head start: everything you do to promote your own emotional health benefits your children—and, in fact, everyone around you—too. Your calm and confident parenting will trickle down calm and confidence to the whole family.

4

SLEEP WELL

Well before I had kids, I was famous in my circle of friends for *needing* my sleep. If I didn't get my eight hours, I was a mess. My friends like to needle me about this—medical school was not full of people sleeping a lot—but the benefits were so clear to me, and the results of lack of sleep so dire for me, that I always kept sleep a priority, no matter what.

My friends who already had kids warned me to say goodbye to all that when I have kids. *Get used to no* sleep, they said. *You'll never have a good night's sleep again*, they said.

I could not imagine how I was ever going to make that work.

When I first became a mom, I learned you just do it.

You don't sleep much. You run on empty. I think the love and excitement and joy somehow keep you (kind of) awake.

This is not a sustainable way to live, though. It doesn't take long for the lack of sleep to catch up to you. This is one of the causes of "mom brain"—the fatigue, the moodiness, the foggy thinking. For plenty of moms, this persists well past when their babies sleep through the night. Between work, kids, and everything else that keeps your life running, it can seem impossible to get a full night's sleep even once, never mind every night.

This is not a setup for calm and confident parenting.

But we already know we need sleep. We know our children need sleep.

We don't always know the *how*.

SLEEP IS GOOD

Sleep—enough of it, and high quality—is crucial for overall health. It promotes heart health, strong immunity, and healthy hormone levels. It regulates metabolism and helps maintain healthy body weight. Sleep (or the lack thereof) also has a big impact on your stress levels, mood, and brain function.

There's a cascade of negative effects when you're not getting enough sleep, too, and they are important enough that figuring out how to make the impossible possible is worth the investment.

The health effects of lack of sleep are significant, including impacting your immune system and therefore increasing susceptibility to infections and illness, increased inflammation, increased risk of weight gain (and the attendant risks of being overweight), and increased risk of heart disease. You'll be more stressed, anxious, distracted, impulsive, and cranky—for both adults and kids.

Health effects show up at the day-to-day level as well. When you're living with chronically insufficient sleep, your food choices get worse, you're a lot less likely to exercise and—you don't need me to tell you this—you'll be impatient and irritable. Lack of sleep, or poor sleep, can increase anxiety as well. What's worse, all this runs in a cycle, and when you're not eating right or getting exercise, it can interfere with sleep and make everything worse.

KIDS' SLEEP

Getting your own rest is key to calm and confident parenting, but so is getting your *kids* good sleep. Sleep strengthens their immune response, helps them maintain a healthy weight, improves their mood, and promotes better learning and attention spans. Kids not getting enough sleep can be cranky, moody, and prone to tantrums. And *you* will find it that much more difficult to be a calm and confident parent in that circumstance.

With enough sleep, consistently, children will be happier and more positive overall.

Just like you.

SLEEP CHANGED HER LIFE

Jana, a friend of a friend, once told me her kid never wanted to go to sleep. She was still a baby, but she never napped during the day. In the evening, she was inconsolable, crying and crying. When the baby didn't sleep, the mom didn't sleep. Jana was beyond exhausted. And so stressed!

Somehow, this hadn't come up with her pediatrician. And Jana, a first-time mom, just thought that babies nap when they get tired. No one had told her parents might have to help set the napping pattern. To me, it was clear her wailing daughter was severely overtired by evening—so overtired she was unable to fall asleep.

Once Jana was let in on the idea of scheduled naps, she grabbed on to the concept immediately. The transition was a bit tricky, because of course it took a while for both her and her daughter to get the hang of something new. But once they did, Jana's whole life changed. She was showering! Running errands! Talking with friends! There were so many things she could squeeze in while her daughter napped that had been out of reach before. Most important, though, was that her (well-rested) daughter was much happier. With her stress lifted, a little time to get things done, and a calmer baby, Jana told me she was like a whole different parent—calmer, happier, and more like herself.

LACK OF SLEEP AND WEIGHT GAIN

Lack of sleep can increase the risk of gaining weight, in adults and kids both. It can make us feel hungrier, crave unhealthy foods, and make poorer food choices. Also, fat cells in the body create a hormone called leptin, which signals us to stop eating. Sleep deprivation decreases the level of this hormone. Our bodies don't get the message we've had enough, so we often just keep eating.

At the same time, lack of sleep increases levels of another hormone, ghrelin. Ghrelin's whole job is to increase your appetite! Of course you are going to eat more when you get hit with higher levels of this hormone.

Over time, all this can lead to weight gain and, therefore, all the associated risks of excess weight.

So the good news is, good sleep helps to maintain a healthy weight—for adults and kids alike.

ENDING SLEEP BATTLES

Another big challenge to calm parenting is the amount of stress so many homes have surrounding bedtime, sleep schedules, or interrupted sleep at night. Getting into a regular routine that ensures a good night's sleep for everyone *can* be done, no matter what's going on in your house right now. Settling everyone into one is a great setup for calm and confident parenting.

Bedtime Chaos

Kids will find every excuse not to go to bed. They are really good at this and will go to great lengths to keep up the effort. Your job is to hold the line anyway, without being sidetracked by frustration or even amusement. The calm and confident approach is simply to stick to a consistent bedtime and establish a strong bedtime routine.

Set a bedtime. Children need different amounts of sleep depending on their age. Watch for a child who is yawning or seems tired early in the day, which are signs they are not getting enough sleep. Watch out, also, for a child who appears awake and hyper at the end of the day. Don't be fooled! This is a sign they are overtired and really need their sleep.

Making bedtime even fifteen to twenty minutes earlier can help, and one way to work out bedtime is to work from when they need to get up in the morning. You also need a bedtime that fits your family schedule. I've been told more than once that my children go to bed "too late." The relevant question is not what the clock says at bedtime. What's important is how many hours of sleep follow. I enjoy the time with them after dinner and into the bedtime routine, hearing about their days, reading together, and so on, and I wasn't getting home from work early enough to have that family time and a 7 p.m. tuck in. And anyway, I don't need them up at 5 a.m.! I know they get an appropriate number of hours of sleep for their ages, and that's what matters to me.

Create a bedtime routine. Routine makes kids feel safe and secure, and the predictability itself helps them relax. Use a bedtime routine to nurture your relationship with your child, taking the time to snuggle, talk about whatever your child is thinking about, and just generally give your undivided attention and show your child you are there for them.

Whatever the components of your routine, make sure it is all calming. Incorporate whatever helps them feel calm and relaxed, like dimmed lights or gentle music. Bedtime book reading is great for both bonding and relaxing, *and* it develops a love of reading. Avoid screens for at least an hour before bed.

Even if bedtime is the furthest thing from calm in your home right now, do not give in and let your child stay up late night after night. If you can avoid making it a full-blown battle and stay calm yourself, a strong routine will do the trick in most cases. (Give it a little time to become a habit.) It may not always be easy to hold the bedtime line, but it is totally worth it!

Child Sleeping in Mom's Bed

This may or may not have been your choice at some point, but now you want your child to sleep in their own bed. The way to approach this: slowly. Let your child know they are going to have their own bed and that you are going to be there for them as they learn how. Stay near them as they fall asleep, initially. Leave the light on if they prefer. Find that special doll or stuffed animal that's a comfort to your child. Keep the night routine the same as it has been—now's not the time to change up anything else.

If your child wakes in the night and comes back to your bed, bring them back to their own right away. Stay with them as they fall back to sleep, but not indefinitely.

Sleep Routine Disrupted

Whatever the reason behind it, when a sleep routine gets disrupted, it is hard on everybody. There's moodiness and crankiness—and not just in the kids! They'll be tired and need extra love and support. (Likely, so will you.)

BEDTIME SNACK

It's a familiar story: the child not hungry at dinner time is starving, they insist, at bedtime. Eating too close to bedtime, or eating too much, can disrupt sleep. But so will feeling hungry. So, try offering a snack about an hour before bed. (Or even closer to bedtime if your child says they are hungry.) Obviously stay away from foods high in sugar, which will keep them up. Try foods high in tryptophan, which helps with sleep. Try dairy as a pro-sleep snack, or nuts or seeds. For my kids, I like to combine that with some carbs, like a few whole-wheat crackers.

If sleep is disrupted because of teething, illness, or travel, give that extra support, and plenty of it, but trust that your child will adjust back to their normal sleep schedule with time—and usually, rather quickly.

If a time change is the issue, you have a chance to get ahead of the curve. About a week before the clocks change, start to put your child to bed ten minutes earlier each night (when you're preparing to "spring ahead"). This way, your child will gradually get used to falling asleep at the regularly scheduled time. It beats trying to get your child to go to bed a whole hour early the day of the change! Throughout the process, stick to the usual routine for getting ready for bed and falling asleep. If you have darkening shades, use them to prevent your child from feeling like they are going to bed while it is still light outside. Fortunately, our bodies like schedule and routine and will quickly adapt to this kind of shift—usually after no more than a week.

If a vacation is the cause of the disruption, whether you've traveled across time zones or have just moved too far away from the usual bedtime routine, you have to make some repairs. Do take preventative measures as you can. For example, if your child still naps at home, plan to allow for those naps.

If you are crossing time zones, consider just keeping your child on your local *home* time for bedtime. Keeping them awake to get them to local vacation time doesn't always work. In fact, children can get so overtired and rundown they don't want to sleep at all, and that's not going to make travel fun. Upon your return from vacation, keep nap and bedtime routines the same, with emphasis on quiet time and calming activities near bedtime. Expect some overnight awakenings the first few days back, and maybe longer-than-normal naps during the day. As with time changes, bodies like schedules and will adjust with time.

"Bad Dreams"

When your child wakes in the middle of the night crying or scared, it can be difficult to remain calm and confident yourself. Nightmares are bad enough, but I will never forget my child's night terrors and how upsetting those episodes were.

To best help your child with these issues, figure out how to stay calm and confident yourself. Start by understanding what is going on so you can react appropriately (hint: it's different for nightmares than it is for night terrors). Then look for the most likely causes—addressing those provides your best bet for reducing recurrence.

Nightmares are very common, especially in preschool children, as they start to have great imaginations. They occur in the later part of the night, after a child has been sleeping for a while, and during the REM stage of sleep.

When your child has a nightmare, hug and comfort them. Provide reassurance it was just a dream and is not real, and that everyone is home and safe. Remind your child where they can find you if they need anything so they can get comfortable going back to sleep. Basically, do just as your mom instinct would tell you to do! The next day, you can talk about the dream, if your child is willing and able. Talking it over (in the morning) can be especially helpful if a particular dream is recurring.

Nightmares can be caused by any stress or change. Often, they are about whatever is going on in the child's life at that time. Sometimes, though, there just is no "reason" at all. So to prevent nightmares, to the degree possible, keep an eye on stress (see Chapter 3 on emotional health), make sure bedtime is peaceful, calm, routinized, and on time, avoid any triggers you can identify, and set them up for a good night's sleep—make sure they have a favorite stuffed animal, and do whatever else is relaxing for them.

Night terrors may be similarly disruptive of the household's sleep, but they're a whole different ball game. They are also much less common. They occur early on in the night after your child goes to sleep, during a non-REM deep stage of sleep. Your child won't remember having a night terror because they are not really awake when they occur (even though it can seem as if they are).

Because they are still asleep, even if they are sitting up and crying or screaming, you will not be able to console a child with night terrors. This is really difficult for a parent to witness. Even so, it is best not to wake them—it would be difficult to, anyway, and also may make it take longer for them to go back to sleep.

Typically a child with night terrors will return to calm sleep quickly, even within minutes, and usually after not more than thirty minutes. It might take you longer to calm yourself back down!

Just know that your child is okay and will be fine, even though it is upsetting to see while it is happening. Remind yourself that they won't remember what happened and that when you are able to help them settle back down to calm sleep, you have done a good job. Most cases of night terrors resolve on their own and are not cause for concern.

You may be able to help prevent recurrence though, or at least some recurrences. Night terrors are more likely to occur when a child is overtired, or is under stress, such as an illness or being in a new environment. Reduce stress as best you can, keep a bedtime routine, and keep your child well rested. Even just going to bed fifteen minutes earlier can be enough to make a difference for some kids with night terrors.

If anyone other than yourself ever cares for your child any time they are asleep, make sure to let them know about the night terrors and how to handle them if they occur.

GOOD QUALITY AND QUANTITY SLEEP

Kids aren't the only ones who benefit from good habits around going to sleep. Adults need seven to nine hours of sleep per night, though most of us don't get it. An occasional five-hour night is okay; you'll function the next day—but your body can't sustain that. I want to urge you to make this a priority for yourself. It's a big ask for busy moms, I know. But it is that important—and it *is* possible. And I say that fully familiar with the way those hours after the children are asleep are your chance to get everything done *and* your chance to have a little downtime to yourself. I'm saying, sleep is so important, it is more important than even those things. And come on, who doesn't love sleeping?

Prioritizing sleep (for you) is the first—and a giant—step. It's a challenge for busy mom's, but here are some ways to make a good night's sleep a regular reality for you (and just know, I'll talk more about fitting in all this in later chapters):

Set a healthy sleep-wake cycle. Aim to fall asleep and wake up at about the same times each day, beginning by going to bed at the same time each night. If you need time to wind down before you fall asleep, go to bed early enough to allow time for that. Going to bed early leaves you time to relax without getting anxious that you are not able to sleep, which only worsens any other anxiety you may be feeling and can keep you up.

Schedule your wake-up time to be consistent from day to day—try not to sleep in. Your body will get used to that quickly. It likes the consistency.

Be physically active each day. Exercise does a lot of good things for you, including promoting good sleep. Getting exercise will help you fall asleep faster, stay asleep, and get a better quality of sleep. It also can reduce insomnia by decreasing stress and anxiety and affecting your circadian rhythm (the body's internal clock) in ways that support sleep.

Cut out evening caffeine. Even afternoon caffeine can interfere with good sleep.

Limit alcohol, which, in excess, can disrupt the quality and quantity of your sleep.

Stick to a healthy diet. A diet high in sugar, fat, or processed foods can interfere with your sleep. Foods your body has a hard time digesting can also keep you up.

Shut off electronics at least an hour before bedtime. The added stimulus, and even the particular kind of light emitted, can keep you awake.

Quiet the mind. Set the mood for a good night's rest by avoiding overstimulation near bedtime. An hour or so before, keep the lights low, read or listen to music, or do other activities you enjoy and find relaxing. Some people find it calming to make lists for the next day or otherwise organize their thoughts as a way to eliminate some stress. Whatever it is that calms you, do that.

Try mindfulness meditation. Some people find they are more successful with meditation right before bed because it is a quieter part of the day and they are not rushing to be going anywhere. Even just ten to twenty minutes before bed can help reduce stress and improve sleep. There are some great apps to try, including many with guidance specifically related to sleep. There are many choices, so you can ask friends for recommendations or just try a few different ones to figure out what works best for you.

Control humidity in the bedroom. Humidity that's too high is uncomfortable enough to disrupt sleep. Too sweaty? Try a dehumidifier. Air conditioners also work by decreasing humidity, so you can try running one, even if on low. Cotton PJs can help you feel less sticky.

Humidity that's too low can lead to a dry, scratchy, itchy throat and sometimes nasal irritation and even nosebleed. A humidifier is great, especially in the wintertime. Or just leaving out a bowlful of water can add moisture to the air.

DO IT ANYWAY

Parenthood makes getting good sleep a challenge, but figuring out how to sleep well is crucial to your parenting experience and performance. Give yourself permission to make it a priority. You need good sleep, and plenty of it. You deserve it. You can do it!

5

EAT WELL

One of my proudest moments in parenting occurred on a night I'd been scrambling to get dinner on the table because my kids were *starving, Mom!* We'd finally sat down and began digging in when my children noticed, *Where are the vegetables?* I'd been pretty happy with a plate of chicken and rice, apparently, but my kids? No. This was obviously an incomplete meal.

Not to worry, The Night There Were No Vegetables turned out to be an emergency of extremely short duration. The asparagus was still on the cooling stove, where I'd somehow overlooked it while serving out our plates.

Kids in general get a bad rap as picky eaters. While truly limited eating is a real and bothersome thing in some cases, the truth is that most kids willingly eat—even demand!—their veggies, as well as a wide variety of other foods sometimes dismissed as "for grownups."

Mine love salmon, quinoa, and cauliflower "rice," and yours can too. If kids are eating their meals with grownups who enjoy their veggies, and veggies are always a matter-of-fact part of family meals, then when the asparagus *isn't* on the table—you're going to hear about it. Like so much else about caring for kids, the secret is to take good care of yourself first, and in this case, that means eating right, including all kinds of healthy foods.

Of course, I know a lot of moms who feel they are just too busy to possibly eat right. Or that when it comes to healthy eating, it's all they can do to focus on their children's nutrition, and they somehow subsist on coffee, what the kids leave on their plates, and whatever they can grab and get down *fast*. Or, feeling so tired, they often eat as essentially a staying-awake strategy—not a setup for great food choices.

I'm here to tell you it is *not* impossible to eat well.

It is, in fact, entirely possible.

You can get your kids to eat healthy foods, feed yourself just as well as you feed them, instill lifelong positive habits in them, and model your own healthy choices. Yes, even when you think there is not even one more minute in the day to devote to meal prep.

And when you do, you are not only going to reap the benefits to your own health, you are going to be much better positioned to parent positively. Your kids are going to benefit not only from the good nutrition but also from a healthier mom who is optimizing her parenting game.

You can do all this while putting an end to the short-order cook method of preparing separate meals for every person. No more mealtime power struggles. Think how much calmer your parenting life will be from these changes alone!

TROUBLE AT THE TABLE

Many moms spend a lot of attention and energy on their children's diets. Healthy eating habits for kids is a great hashtag mom-goal, but a less healthy pattern for themselves often comes right alongside these good intentions. That is, moms' concerns for what their kids eat takes up so much space, ensuring excellent nutrition *for themselves* seems to go right out the window!

A healthy diet is not only key to maintaining your weight but also to all aspects of your physical, mental, and emotional well-being. A poor diet has been linked to being overweight or obese, as well as to high blood pressure, high cholesterol, heart disease, depression, and more. What I want to call particular attention to, though, is the way eating poorly affects your parenting. (Hint: it doesn't make it better!) Prioritizing your own good nutrition is a key part of the foundation for calm and confident parenting.

I'm going to give you more detailed plans for how to pull this off later in the chapter, but here's the most basic secret to how it works: eat what your kids eat. Or, if you prefer, serve your kids what you serve yourself.

No need for either of you to consume "nuggets" of anything. And—you may have to trust me on this, at first—no need for you to forgo the healthy pleasures of roasted brussels sprouts or mashed sweet potato. Your kids can and will develop a taste for them, just as you have. This is, in fact, a gift to them that they will carry into their adult lives. You will be a great role model for healthy eating— and they will do what kids always do: learn by watching what their parents do. Don't let the lesson be *I'm too busy for anything but processed or unhealthy foods.* Let them see you nourish yourself well and enjoying your food every day.

TOO TIRED TO EAT RIGHT

Moms are often caught in a vicious cycle of eating poorly, which leads to feeling tired and fatigued and having low energy—which leads to more eating poorly. Being overweight can also cause fatigue, compounding the problems.

None of that is good. But there's an even more problematic effect here: the fatigue and the not-great eating both impact your mood and your ability to be patient and present for your kids. Poor nutrition will curb your ability to parent calmly and confidently, just when you need it most!

This whole cycle might kick off from the sleep-deprived state many parents exist in, or from some other situation that gets back-burnered after taking care of the kids.

For me, it was a sports injury that caused a whole breakdown in the way I was used to eating. Which happened while I was pregnant with my second child! My usual workouts—already squished in however I could manage them as a working mom—were interrupted, and that wasn't doing any favors to my energy levels or mood. I felt tired all the time, and sluggish. As tired as I was, I was eating more to try to stay awake and craving the most sugary, least healthy foods more and more. Making a whole well-rounded dinner seemed like just too much some days, and I was eating whatever on-the-go food I could pick up; most of it was not particularly healthy. And, wouldn't you know, this way of eating was combining with the decreased exercise to disturb my sleep. Just when I thought I couldn't feel more fatigued…I did.

LACK OF SLEEP MAKES YOU OVEREAT

One of my top "diet" tips is to do what you need to do to get a good night's sleep every night. It's at least as important as exercise for maintaining a healthy weight. Lack of sleep, and the resulting fatigue, increases the risk of gaining weight and overeating. It also disrupts the hormones regulating appetite and your hunger cues.

Have you noticed that when you get tired you eat more? Or that you eat more, or "cheat" more, toward the end of the day, when you are more fatigued? Or that your willpower decreases with your energy levels?

The science backs up your observation. For example, one study showed people sleeping less than four hours a night eat more than 22 percent more calories per day. That's going to add up. Even as parents, most of us can manage more than four hours sleep a night, but any amount of sleep deprivation can alter your appetite and metabolism enough to cause weight gain.

Eventually, I recognized the pattern that was staring me in the face: the worse I ate, the more tired I felt, and the more tired I felt, the worse I ate. As my injury healed, I was able to get back in a healthier groove. This natural experiment made a big impact on me, and I won't soon forget its lessons about how the way I was eating and feeling impacted my ability to parent the way I wanted to parent.

QUICK STRATEGIES TO GET STARTED

So, what is a busy mom to do? It can seem impossible to

eat right when there's so little time and so much on your plate! A few basic strategies will help you feed yourself and your kids the healthy foods you need to fuel your busy lives:

- Schedule meal planning time once or twice a week—as well as a coordinated grocery shopping time. If you don't plan out your meals (and shopping), you won't have what you need on hand to create healthy meals efficiently. And you'll end up always on the go and grabbing less healthy options along the way. Not only will you end up with poorer quality food that way, in both nutrition and taste, but you will also lose track of the quantity of food you eat.
- Plan quick, simple, well-balanced meals. Remember, family dinners do not need to be extravagant or in any way Instagram-worthy. My meals are so the opposite! Still, my kids have been known to declare a plate of basic salmon, sweet potato, and brussels sprouts "the best meal ever!" Turns out my kids don't follow any Instagram influencers, and they don't know that some moms arrange every vegetable into animal shapes or otherwise fancy it up.
- Stock the refrigerator, freezer, and pantry with healthy options for snacks and for easy meals. And *don't* stock unhealthy items that will be especially tempting when you are short on time or low on energy.
- Make home-cooked meals your standard option, and

don't rely on takeout or restaurant meals. They are never as healthy as what you make at home and are pretty much guaranteed to be in larger portions.
- Make sure everyone drinks plenty of water. You'd be surprised how much difference that makes to your energy levels, hunger signals, and mood.
- Pack snacks ahead of time, for you and the kids. That makes it easy to grab appealing options even when you're running out. It's just as convenient for making sure snacks at home are fresh, tasty, healthy, and portion-controlled. Don't be the mom who carries healthy snacks for the kids then grabs whatever junky snack she can find for herself!

MAKE TIME FOR MEAL PREP

I admit I sometimes dread meal prep. But I do it anyway because it actually makes my life so much easier. In fact, it makes the eating-healthy-homecooked-meals thing even possible. Otherwise, it's back to the days when my kids get home from after-school activities and within minutes are complaining they are starving—and me with no way to get dinner on the table fast enough to avoid meltdowns or poor-quality snacks. I've had enough of those experiences to last me, thank you very much. I'm grateful to myself pretty much every day when I pull out what I've prepped.

I find prepping twice a week works best. For me, Sunday and

Wednesday turn out to be easier than doing twice as much on Sunday—and it also allows for fresher options. I don't want to leave raw fish sitting around all week, waiting for its turn! An exception is all the nonperishable snacks. I do those in one go over the weekend, for both the kids and me.

You will find the system that works best for you. Just *having* a system in place is what matters. That's what keeps you on track.

STRESS AND EATING

Just in case you ever find mom life stressful (ha!), let's look at the connections between stress and eating. We already know how stress can create a powerful urge for comfort foods—most of which are not from the healthiest sections of the menu. There's a physical component to this: stress increases hormones in a way that can trigger food cravings for sugar, salt, and fatty foods. Of course stress can also lead to emotional eating—or "eating your feelings."

These patterns hold for both parents and kids. In fact, it is especially important to watch for signs of emotional eating in young children, or anyone who may not always have the words to express themselves. It doesn't have to be from any great wave of emotion, either—probably the most common pattern, in adults and kids, is eating out of boredom.

It's normal, and okay, to want the occasional extra snack or unhealthier option, and in moderation this is exactly what a "treat" is. But you don't want this to become a regular way to deal with your emotions. Eating is not a workable—or effective—emotional regulation strategy over time.

In addition, poor nutrition is physical stress on the body. It is a stress with a straightforward solution. Eating right supports optimal well-being—mentally, physically, and emotionally. When are you more likely to make great parenting moves—while running on coffee and a doughnut or two by mid-afternoon, or after you've had eggs for breakfast, your favorite salad for lunch, and a go-to stash of almonds stowed in your purse?

In stressful times, it is helpful to stick to a routine as much as possible, especially when it comes to meals and snacks. Follow a schedule for three regular meals, and healthy, planned snacks—for adults and kids alike. This should eliminate hunger pangs and reduce mindless snacking, which usually results in less healthy choices that are less nutrient-dense.

Of course, this plan relies on you planning for and stocking healthy options. I also advise eating in a designated eating area, like the kitchen table, at least when you are at home.

These are practical strategies that will work to contain mindless eating, but even better, of course, is to address the underlying stress or emotional triggers. This can be as simple as distracting a bored child with an activity rather than a snack. But sometimes it requires a more involved intervention.

Whatever approaches you decide on, short and long term, perhaps the most important component is to learn to listen to your body and its cues about when it is full and when it is hungry. Eating all the time—"grazing"—can prevent you and/or your child from noticing hunger cues, and knowing when you are actually hungry and when you are not. That's a recipe for overeating. The adult version is often rushing around and eating on the go and eating so quickly that you don't have time to assess when you are actually full. Or, eating when food is available, whether or not you are hungry, because who knows when you will get another chance to eat? (Hint: if you have a healthy snack ready to go, and with you…you'll know.)

HEALTHY ADULTHOOD STARTS IN CHILDHOOD

Childhood obesity is on the rise nationally. Nearly one in three kids are overweight already, with rates still climbing—and those rates increase as kids get older! A recent statistic predicted *more than half* of two-year-olds will be obese by the time they are thirty-five. This is not great, and it gets worse: overweight and obese kids are more likely to be overweight or obese in adulthood, and as we know, being overweight is a risk factor for diabetes and cardiovascular disease, and for experiencing those at younger ages.

Interrupting this pattern gets harder as kids get older, so it is important to instill healthy eating habits young—the earlier, the better. By the time a child is six or seven, it is more difficult to reverse negative habits and their effects. Prevention must be the priority. (The younger your kids start exposure to healthy eating, the better, so allow me one overall note of caution: as with any food, be aware of potential choking hazards, especially for toddlers, and avoid or prepare foods accordingly.)

It is, however, never too late. Raising kids to be healthy is a long-term project. And it's small changes that will add up to big differences for you and your family. For example, teach your children that it is okay not to clean their plates. If they are not hungry for all of it, don't force or cajole them into eating all of it. Maybe add one more home-cooked meal per week. Or one more veggie to the typical day's menu. Start wherever you are, and improve from there.

Obesity rates are increasing in kids for lots of the same reasons they are increasing in adults: insufficient exercise/movement, unhealthy foods, poor portion control, eating despite bodily cues that you are not hungry, and eating out of boredom, or for emotional or social reasons. Still, the combination of eating right, moving your body, and getting sufficient, high-quality sleep provides a workable solution. You are modeling healthy eating habits.

Eating right matters to you and to your kid and to your kid's future.

Discussing with your children what it feels like to be hungry and full matters. Teaching your children to listen to their bodies, including how to tell the difference between hunger and boredom, sadness, or tiredness, matters. Just don't expect your child to practice any of this if you don't.

"MY KIDS WON'T EAT THIS WAY"

I think we've all agreed that starting a healthy diet in the early years helps your children launch toward healthy adulthood—surely, a key parenting goal.

But what if your kid won't eat healthy food? This is the number one objection I hear from parents. They can hardly even imagine a bite of broccoli passing their kids' lips. Salmon? Forget about it! *May*be a few blueberries…

But it's a misconception. Kids will eat great, nutritious foods. They'll *like* them. Love them even.

(The second most common objection I hear from moms is that they don't have time to create and serve healthy menus all day every day. Also not true! We'll get there.)

It's true not every kid comes out of the womb loving brussels sprouts and black beans, but most can and do appreciate many healthy, tasty foods. It just might take some practice. Like anything else, eating healthy can take getting used to. It might also require some smooth parenting.

SERVE (AND EAT) HEALTHY FOODS

The first thing to do is to serve the foods you want your kids to eat. And eat them. Everyone gets the same meals. The upcoming superfoods section has lots of ideas about which ones and ways to serve them.

If your child refuses a food, don't make a big deal out of it. But *do* keep offering it, and maybe make it different ways. They may like it next time! Or the time after that, or…

It can take multiple tries of a new food before your child accepts it into their repertoire. Toddlers, especially, can be very picky, so bring your patience. At whatever age, the important thing is to keep introducing new foods, in small amounts, one at a time—and to repeat way more times than you probably think is reasonable.

TRY THIS PIZZA

My son loooooooves pizza (I know, surprise!) but outright rejected the very idea of a cauliflower pizza crust. My mistake might have been putting a name to it too soon. When I brought home a new kind of pizza, he agreed to give it a try: pizza is pizza. He soon declared his love for it.

When I said, "Oh, yay!" he got suspicious.

"Mommy, is this cauliflower pizza?" I confessed it was. I wasn't out to trick him, really, just to allow an open mind. But then, the miracle happened: "I like it better than regular."

Not a miracle that he'd like it, or try it...but a miracle that he'd admit he liked it after the definitive pronouncements he'd made about the validity of cauliflower crust! Kids like all kinds of healthy foods, and yours can too.

As long as they are not grazing all day, kids will be hungry at the start of a meal, which makes this great timing for trying a new veggie or a new preparation or a new dish. *You like mashed sweet potato, now how about this lovely chunk of roasted sweet potato, skin and all?*

You do want to find the foods your kids actually like. This is not about wearing down wary eaters until they eat something just to get it over with. Everyone prefers some foods over others, and prefers to avoid some altogether. And all that is fine—as long as in the big picture there are a variety of good foods on the list.

You *don't* want trying new foods to become another time-consuming stressor. Encourage new foods as often as you can, and keep trying, but don't let this become a battle.

Praise your kids any time they try a food, but don't give any reward just for eating. You don't want your child to expect—or hold out for—a toy or treat because they ate the same carrots today they happily wolfed down yesterday. Enjoying a good food, even a healthy food, is its own reward for kids just like it is for you.

PROVIDE PLENTY OF CHOICES

Strategy number two is to present your kids with options. Let them choose which healthy foods they want for meals and snacks. Ask them what they want when you are meal planning. Take them to the grocery store with you and offer them healthy choices for them to choose between. *Should we get turkey burgers or veggie burgers?*

Have them pick out at least one vegetable and at least one fruit. At home, let them choose what's on the menu. Even the choice between which of the foods they picked out that they have on which days will help them feel more in control. Kids will eat what they have chosen. Give them choices!

The quality of the meals you eat will be higher since, remember, you are eating the same food as your children.

And as a bonus, this upfront investment will save time and conflict in the end.

CREATE EXCITEMENT ABOUT HEALTHY FOOD

Getting kids excited about foods is the best way to get them to try and like (most of) them. Letting them help you prepare foods—everything from filling up snack bags to making the menu to determining the preparation of a side dish to tossing the dinner salad—is a great way to build that excitement. Kids will eat what they have cooked or even just dished out, like taking baby carrots out of the baggie themselves and spooning yogurt dip on the plate next to them.

Get creative about how you give your kids foods. Mixing veggies into foods they already love can help. I wouldn't "hide" them, or how will they know what they liked and would like more of, in different ways? (Plus, who's got time to purée beets just to mix them into something else so complicated they are undetectable?) But maybe throw some peas in the (whole grain) pasta they already devour.

Try different varieties of a food too. *You like applesauce, how about this apple?* And then, *You like this red delicious apple, how about this crunchy, tart green apple?* Or even, *You like apples, how about apples mixed in with roasted root vegetables?*

Try different preparations: after roasted root veggies with apples, how about *puréed* roasted root veggies with apples? Or vice versa. *If you love broccoli dusted with Parmesan, how about brussels sprouts served that way?*

SUPERFOODS MOST KIDS LOVE

OK, but what *exactly* am I supposed to get my kid to eat?

You and your children need the same things out of your diet: complex carbohydrates, protein, healthy fats, and vitamins and minerals—sourced, as much as possible, from vegetables, fruits, and whole grains.

You can fast-track your family to an overall healthy diet by including plenty of whole, nutrient-dense foods in your everyday lives. These are so-called superfoods, packed with nutrients including antioxidants, vitamins, and minerals.

Your freshest choices will vary seasonally, and there are many more than this list to choose from, but here are my top picks:

- Blueberries. Fresh berries are great first finger foods. Freezing berries—or really, small pieces of any fruit—adds magical appeal to most kids. Stirring berries into yogurt is also a popular pick.
- Sweet potato. Bake or steam as is. Mash for babies, on

its own, or added in cereal. If for some reason the natural sweetness doesn't immediately captivate your child, there's always sweet potato fries to make the case for you!
- Broccoli. Purée for babies—or add some purée to mac and cheese or any pasta dish.
- Spinach. Purée for younger kids who are skeptical.
- Brussels sprouts. Sprinkle some Parmesan over them and roast/bake in the oven until browned and softened. Some kids like to dip in ketchup.
- Cauliflower. Just steamed plain is good, or treat like the brussels sprouts above. Mash or purée cauliflower for babies or younger children—though grownups may love it this way too!
- Oatmeal. Add raisins, cinnamon, or honey to increase interest. (Remember that honey is not for babies younger than one year old.)
- Kale. Two words: kale chips. Simply coat clean, dry kale leaves with some olive oil and bake. You might add a very light sprinkle of salt, but try them plain first. Crispy, healthy chips—what's not to love?!
- Winter squash. Most babies love puréed winter squash thanks to its natural sweetness…and grownups usually do too! Add some cinnamon for extra flavor.
- Spaghetti squash. Roast, and then scrape out the strands. Many people love it served just like its namesake pasta, with red sauce. But if this strikes your kids as a poor substitute, try other preparations you might use with noodles, like pesto or olive oil and garlic.

- Asparagus. Nothing beats plain grilled asparagus with just a little olive oil. My kids also love it just steamed.
- Dates. These make a great dessert, on their own, or added to baked goods. Remove pit from date for young children, and break into very small pieces.

And, don't forget these superfood proteins kids love:

- Nuts—especially almonds, my favorite snack. Some kids prefer nut butters to whole nuts.
- Eggs. Kids usually like scrambled eggs as soon as they move past an all-puree diet.
- Salmon. My kids love it plain grilled, just like me. If your kids are still learning to like salmon, try it in a pasta dish or made into a "salad" with mayo.
- Greek yogurt. Add fruit to plain yogurt to avoid added sugars, which are usually very high in flavored yogurts. For a "treat and trick," stir blueberries or other fruit into vanilla Greek yogurt and use it to fill cupcake liners. Maybe sprinkle a little granola or mini chocolate chips on the top or bottom. Freeze two to three hours until firm. It looks like a cupcake and tastes like ice cream!
- Edamame. Most kids love these, especially when they get to pop them out of the pods themselves. Food you can play with! Make sure young kids eat these sitting down to avoid any choking risk from unchewed beans.

INFLAMMATORY FOODS

For overall health, try to avoid inflammatory foods.

Most common foods to limit to avoid inflammation:

- Sugars, including soda, candy, and baked goods.
- Artificial sweeteners, which can trigger unwanted immune responses.
- Refined flour, as in white breads and traditional pizza crusts and pastas, which can cause inflammation. Choose whole grain options instead. They will keep you feeling fuller, longer, too!
- Red meat, when it gives your body excess saturated fat, increases inflammation. Stick to one serving a week if you include it in your diet.
- "Bad" fats, especially partially hydrogenated oils. Avoid fried foods because they are usually made with partially hydrogenated oils. As above, limit saturated fats, as found in meats, cheese, butter, and cream. The tricky part: coconut oil is a saturated fat, but it has *anti*-inflammatory properties!
- Imbalanced amounts of vegetable oils and their omega-6 fatty acids. You need some of these fats, as found in sunflower, safflower, corn, canola, and other vegetable oils, but we tend to get amounts way out of proportion to anti-inflammatory omega-*3* fatty acids (as in oily fish). Such an imbalance may cause inflammation, so your best bet is to stick to olive oil, with

its anti-inflammatory properties and healthy monounsaturated fats.

ANTI-INFLAMMATORY FOODS

Many of my favorite *anti*-inflammatory foods are choices your children will love too. I don't know too many kids who will pass up berries and chocolate!

- Broccoli.
- Avocado.
- Green tea.
- Turmeric.
- Berries. Blueberries may be the most famously healthy, but strawberries, blackberries, and raspberries are all great (and popular) choices.
- Extra virgin olive oil.
- Fatty fish. I remember which fish are great sources of omega-3s with the acronym SMASH—salmon, mackerel, anchovies, sardines, and herring.
- Dark chocolate

EAT IT UP

Getting the whole family to eat well is a major parenting challenge—and doing so successfully is a major boon for your parenting. Make healthy food choices an unremarkable part of every family meal and regular family life, and then you'll be the one with stories to tell about kids asking, *Where are the vegetables?!*

6

KEEP MOVING

I've done a lot of experimenting on the effects of exercise, with myself as the test subject. These may not be the sort of trials that you would submit for peer review or get published in a journal, but I've gotten enough data to convince me it has a major impact on all aspects of my health—and sanity!

Most recently, a stress fracture in my foot required me to take time off from my usual workouts. I'd been doing some fitness activity pretty much every day—maybe not for very long each day, but enough. With the stress fracture, I had to stop cold turkey for a while as I figured out what I could do and enjoy (and fit in) that didn't put pressure on that foot.

It wasn't long before I noticed I felt tired and sluggish all the time. I began making less healthy choices with my food and was not up to any extra effort to eat healthily. And I found myself snacking mindlessly in an attempt to feel more awake—mostly high-sugar foods, of course. Despite feeling tired, I began sleeping poorly, likely from the combination of poor diet and lack of exercise. That, of course, did less than nothing to alleviate my fatigue. I also noticed the lack of sleep affecting my mood. I definitely became more tense and less patient with my kids.

Gradually, I found ways to keep moving while protecting my foot, and when the doctor finally cleared me to resume my favorite activities, the difference was immediate and profound. I saw change right away as I got back into a routine of spending some time each day working out. It may have been only about twenty minutes, but that was enough to improve my sleep, mood, and energy dramatically. I soon felt like myself again. I had more energy, was more patient, and started eating better.

The same thing happened when I was recovering from my C-section (when I was, of course, also a new mom), and when I broke my foot during my second pregnancy. And when I injured my knee. Oh, and the time I overdid it at my first fitness competition and had to lay off running to let an ankle heal up. And after a hand fracture and surgery...

I may be the only participant in my fitness experiment, but I've replicated my results more times than I care to remember!

I am not the only one who, with regular exercise, will be healthier and make healthier choices. More importantly, I am also not the only one for whom this is the key to being a calmer, happier person and a better parent.

THE BEST MOOD BOOSTER

Of course there's plenty of actual science to back me up on the impacts of fitness on not just physical health but on emotional health as well. Exercise reduces stress and anxiety, keeps your mind active and healthy, and makes you feel better emotionally. Exercise is for sure the best mood booster. Physical activity improves mood overall, helps promote good quality sleep, and produces endorphins that make you feel good in the moment. Doing exercise you really enjoy brings positivity into any day—especially when you are feeling overwhelmed.

With regular exercise, you'll feel more energized, mentally focused, and alert. This makes any exercise you do important not only to you but to everyone around you. With regular exercise, you are going to feel better and be healthier.

DRINK

I want to add one more pillar to your plan for wellness. Simple as it may seem, it ranks right up there with exercise, diet, and sleep when it comes to being healthy: stay well hydrated.

Drinking water, and plenty of it, might be the easiest, most effective single thing you can do for your health.

During a workout is a great time to focus on how much water you're getting—you definitely need it then, and it's an easy time to remember because you'll get clear signs from your body that it wants water. But you need water just as much when you're sitting at your desk or commuting as you do when you're doing a fitness video and taking a run. Aim to keep your water intake up all throughout the day.

PRIORITIZE EXERCISE

We know we need to prioritize fitness activities for ourselves, but for a busy mom, it isn't always obvious how. The first step is just making it a priority. From there, try these strategies.

SCHEDULE YOUR WORKOUTS

Aim for at least twenty minutes of something every day. Something as simple as putting it on your calendar or setting a reminder can solve the "*When do I have time to exercise?*" problem. My experience is, we don't have time because we don't make time.

I set my alarm to be up before my kids to make sure I

get in my twenty-minute workout (more about that to come). But if I don't have an appointment with myself to do this, it's easy for me to waste that time scrolling social media or to put it off for "later," which becomes the next day, and then the next day… Once you miss one day, it's much easier to let the second one go by, and ultimately it's been weeks and you haven't done anything. Block out the time on your schedule and commit to it like any work meeting or other priority.

Schedule both how many days a week you plan on working out and the specific time each day.

THE BEST TIMING FOR YOU

I find mornings are best for exercise. It's a great way to wake yourself up, physically and emotionally, and jump-start the day. It clears your mind, wakes up your brain so you are more mentally alert, boosts your metabolism, regulates your appetite, and makes you feel energized and increases the amount of energy you have for the whole day.

I admit it can be difficult to get out of bed earlier, but I know I always feel better after a workout, and it is so worth it. I love my morning workouts. It changes the whole day for me. I always say morning exercise is my caffeine. I don't drink coffee or any caffeinated beverages—and I don't need to!

Later in the day, something always comes up to derail exercise plans—missed bus, last-minute meeting…or you just get tired from your day. It's never hard to find an excuse. So I find it's best to just fit it in before the rest of your day really takes off.

Exercise in the morning also adds positivity to the start of the day. The endorphins get going, and you get the feeling of having already accomplished something for the day. Your energy is lifted, your mood is lifted, and whatever else has to get done or be dealt with that day seems less daunting. I know it can be tempting to just hit the snooze button instead, but think of it this way: you will probably still feel tired even if you get that fifteen more minutes of sleep. But fifteen minutes of moving your body will definitely make you feel more awake!

If mornings don't work for you, the important thing is really to find what timing is best—which will vary from person to person—and make a regular date with yourself for that time. Note it on your calendar like you would a meeting with a client—and keep it the same way you would if you were doing something for work. Meaning, don't cancel!

Maybe your schedule is more open late in the day. Maybe you like to schedule workouts for times when you are most stressed. In any case, pick your time, but stay flexible too. Expect the unexpected, and be ready to shift when you work out on that day your kids miss the bus or your boss calls you at home before work.

CHANGE EXPECTATIONS

For moms who were into fitness "before kids," what you expect from a workout may have to change. And that's okay. It's okay if you are no longer at the same level of fitness right now. It's okay if you have to switch up your activities for logistical reasons. It's okay if you cut a run short because the baby just spit up (copiously) in the jogging stroller. What matters is doing something you like and fitting it in regularly—with flexibility. Whatever gets your body moving.

Doing what you love is the best way to ensure that you will want to fit exercise into your day. So, go with what you like best. Or keep switching it up until you find what you like best. Or, to help you keep going, maybe doing different things at different times works for you. It's all good—the idea is to enjoy it.

Moms also have to work within the real world, so sometimes what you love most may need to be a really *efficient* workout. If what you like best is running marathons, that's just not going to happen every day, is it? Maybe an hour-and-a-half yoga class with a nice long Shavasana is not going to cut it either.

HIIT ME

You can find any number of HIIT workouts in a few minutes on YouTube or Google, but this is my go-to HIIT workout. It is a series of six exercises you do for 30 seconds each. You can do a full set once or twice to start out, depending on where you are, and increase up to four circuits, which is what I did after my injury.

1. Mountain climbers
2. Plank
3. Squat jumps
4. Standing crunches
5. Burpees
6. Squat punches

The time-crunch problem led me to my current (and longtime) favorite: HIIT, or high-intensity interval training. One routine I use takes just twelve minutes! And the research shows that as far as benefits go, that twelve minutes gives you as much as you'd get from a longer continuous run, in terms of increasing metabolic rate, fat loss, and much more. It's also enough for me to stave off fatigue, feel fit, and stay in a mental state that allows for calm and confident parenting.

Other options for staying in shape on the go can start with the simplest possible combo: sit-ups and pushups; fifteen minutes will do it. If you like running, a short jog around the neighborhood is great, pretty much no matter where you find yourself. Exercise bands and/or small hand weights are very useful at home. And you'll find endless variations on all these, as well as HIIT exercises, with a quick survey of friends or internet search.

EXERCISE WITH YOUR KIDS

There's no need for childcare, no babysitting via screen time, if your kids are working out with you! My kids like to join in with me, at times, when I'm working out at home, and these are not just healthy but also fun and bonding moments. I never force or require this, but when they show interest, I'm always happy to have them play along with me. They may not be doing all the right moves, exactly, but they are moving, we are hanging out, and I am fitting in my workout, so win-win-win.

BE CONSISTENT

I get asked about how I stay fit more than about any other thing, usually with a sense of incredulity that it is even possible for a working single mom with young kids. The real answer is consistency. It matters less what you do, exactly, than that you do it regularly.

People don't always believe me when I say it, but I really love working out. It is my "me" time," and it makes me feel happy. Still, even for me, it sometimes feels like the last thing I want to do. This is especially true when life is at its most chaotic. This is of course also when I most need the stress relief and other benefits that exercise offers.

Here's the truth: starting is the hardest part. I don't really have an easy solution for How to Get Started, but it helps to remember everything else is easier once you do! That can be enough, even on those days of dread, to help you change into your leggings, or get off your phone, or whatever micro-step is in your way.

MARLA IN REAL LIFE

Marla had no time for exercise. She was on the go with her kids from the minute she rolled out of bed. So, yes, she knew exercise was good for her, but let's get real. What was she supposed to cut out to fit in a trip to the gym? Sleep? Making dinner for the family? The half-hour before bed she allowed herself for "me time"? (That was definitely nonnegotiable.) She was exhausted all the time as it was.

The big change for Marla came when she realized she could get a real workout in just twenty minutes, and right at home. And she did have twenty minutes in her day—she spent longer than that on Instagram most days. She could do it while her kids got screen time, as they never budged from their spots while watching videos.

Marla set up a little space in her home, just big enough for her to put down a yoga mat, bookmarked a few short HIIT workout videos her friends recommended, and made her kids' screen time her "gym" time. Now that she's in the groove with this, she hardly misses a day of her five-times-a-week goal. She feels so much better with the regular exercise, from even just these short bursts, that she never really feels like skipping a day.

ARRANGE ACCOUNTABILITY

Get a friend or partner to work out with you—you'll be less likely to cancel when your workout plan includes someone else. Working out with someone might also motivate you to go just a little harder than you would on your own. Even just having someone check in with you about your workouts—someone you have to tell if you skip a day (or week)—can keep you going.

YOUR KID IS JUST LIKE YOU

Physical activity is also important for your kids, of course. They accrue the same physical and emotional benefits as adults—and, often, social benefits as well. Regular exercise will boost moods in kids, too. It's a great way for them to release any anxiety. Just like you, they'll feel less stressed, get better sleep, and have improved focus. These benefits to a child allow a parent to be more readily available to remain calm and confident. That's much easier to do with a non-cranky, well-rested kid!

Encourage your kids to stay physically active by setting your own example. If they see you exercising, working out, and staying fit, they will emulate those habits. They learn the value of fitness and healthy habits in general from observing you. And not just about exercising daily, but also the way you manage your stress and the way you're setting priorities for yourself. Kids are going to see all of that. The messages they absorb about staying healthy, starting very early in their lives, will last into adulthood.

FAMILY FITNESS

There's another way to motivate your children to healthful physical activity that's even more powerful than acting as a role model: family fitness activities. These are a great way to have fun together as a family and create wonderful memories and strengthen family bonds. When you find the right activity for your family that everyone enjoys and is motivated to do, it is the ultimate in quality time.

UNSTRUCTURED PLAY

This is really important for child development. Unstructured activity is just play for kids, and you want to encourage as much of their play as possible to be physical. Extra points for outdoors and/or with friends. This kind of play is great for their motor skills, creativity, social learning, and more.

Plus, the more they are moving around in play, the less they are on a screen. Bonus! And if a kid happens to wear themselves out from jumping in leaves, chasing their pet, or climbing at the playground, and that happens to lead to a good nap or falling asleep early...so much the better, am I right?

Just remember, unstructured play means you don't have much to do with it—except to provide the opportunities to make of their play time what they will. Join in, by all means, but you don't have to. If you do, remember you are not in charge of the activity.

There are many sports you can do as a family, though your choices may change with the age of your children and everyone's interests. My friend Jennifer's family swears by bike riding. When the kids were really little, they may not have gone all that far on each ride, but even with tiny bikes with training wheels, the kids were proud to ride the mile to the duck pond. As the kids have grown, the rides have gotten longer and more challenging, but their enthusiasm has remained.

Maybe you're the family who likes a good game of touch football or can't wait for the ice rink to reopen for the winter. Or maybe hiking is your (collective) thing. Try different things, keep doing what is most enjoyable for you all, and your kids may be getting exercise without even realizing it! Family activities are a great gift to give them—not just for the benefits of exercise but also the attitude that moving your body is a thing you want to do and not just a chore.

Making family fitness a priority from their youngest days and adapting as they grow builds a strong foundation for a lifetime of healthy activity for your children, while keeping you not only healthy but calm and confident in your parenting.

ME AND FITNESS, WE GO WAY BACK

Fitness has always been a big part of my life, going all the way back to high school. At that time, it was all about sports for me, and I played all the way through college.

I always felt better overall with a lot of physical activity in my life. As I got older, I appreciated the mental and emotional benefits more, alongside the physical ones. When I was active, I always felt more awake and stronger in all aspects of my life. It was natural for me to continue to incorporate fitness into my life alongside the business of life—including work, personal things, family, and kids. I made time for it, regardless of what else was happening.

Even when I was a medical resident, post-call and exhausted. Even when I was seven months pregnant with my second child. And even after kids, when it definitely became more challenging to do, but also more necessary than ever. I really rely on that boost of energy from working out and the mood lift that comes with it.

Fitness has been such a powerful positive force in my life—a lesson underscored for me each time I was sidelined from my usual workouts (i.e., learning the hard way). It is possible to fit exercise into even the busiest life. You can do it. In fact, you must.

7

TIME MANAGEMENT, ORGANIZATION, AND ROUTINE

Getting organized in the sense of, "Let's look what is going on in this linen closet, anyway," or, "I'll file when I can no longer see the desktop, thank you" is all well and good. Even more important, though, is getting organized *in your head*. Organize your life as a whole. Organizing bookshelves and cabinets will come, but start with the less concrete, bigger picture. Creating routine and schedules and lists—lots of lists!—and working on time management are all part of the process.

MOM BRAIN

If you, like me, have ever had to turn your home upside down looking for your keys, only to find them in the freezer or still in the door, I don't have to tell you that "mom brain" is absolutely real. You might have mom brain if…you can't quite recall someone's name, or where you left your phone, or how to read a long report without having to go over each paragraph twice.

The feeling of being less mentally clear—less able to focus, just plain forgetful, or like you are in a fog—can last weeks or months after a new child joins the family. I was still using (needing) the excuse I "just" had a baby for years after my kids were born.

Mom brain often follows on top of the similar state known as "pregnancy brain," and in both cases you can thank, from what's actually a long list, hormonal changes, lack of sleep, diet changes, and stress—and the interactions between all these. Scientific evidence shows there are changes in the brain that may cause the forgetfulness associated with early motherhood, and that it is not necessarily due only to the stress and sleep deprivation common to new moms.

So there are self-care approaches to dealing with mom brain (including not judging yourself for something that's this normal and that has origins largely not in your control), and you should definitely practice them. But here's why I'm starting a chapter on time management, organization, and routine with this topic:

First of all, you are busy, really busy. You have a lot of things to do, a lot of directions you are being pulled in, and a finite supply of time and energy. That's not changing anytime soon.

Second, since you are going to have mom brain, you will need to learn how to manage your time, set and maintain a routine, and get and stay organized. You need this so that even when you're a bit fuzzy, even when you have a million things to take care of, and even when the day doesn't go as planned, you don't lose your mind and are happy with your parenting.

Because if you don't already know this, the day is *not* going to go as planned. And if today does, tomorrow's not going to. Things are always going to change. There's going to be some chaos. That's just life—or at least, life with kids. It's always something.

That's not an argument for not making a plan. It's an argument for making *all* the plans. Your watchwords through all of this should be:

1. expect the unexpected,

and

2. be flexible.

For those deep in mom brain territory: "Expect to be flexible."

You make routine and structure and organization *because* things are always going to change. Having a "way you do things" is what allows you to pivot to another way when you need to.

MAKE YOUR BED

I am an inveterate bed maker, and I love that this seems to have been successfully passed to my kids. Even on days when I'm rushing like mad to get out the door, feeling like I have too many things to do to fit into one day, I still always make my bed. It makes me feel calmer, like one small area where I have demonstrated control over my world is a harbinger for the rest of the day.

There are many studies showing the benefits of spending just a few minutes on this one simple task. Making your bed makes you more productive. Completing this small task makes you feel accomplished and encourages you to take another similar step. The most successful people make their beds. Those who make their beds are happier, less stressed, more satisfied with their work life (!), and more likely to maintain a regular exercise routine (!!).

MAKING TIME

The simple fact is that you have so much to do. I know so many moms who worry they will never get everything done and/or won't be able to have the time they want to spend with their kids. They feel as if they have a never-ending to-do list…because they do.

The good news about being so busy and having such limited time is that it makes you extra diligent when it comes to managing what time you do have. Good time management helps you stay on top of all you have to do and increases your efficiency in getting things done. You'll waste less time and decrease your stress and anxiety, enjoying time with your family more and creating more time for yourself. In other words, great time management is a good way to facilitate being a calm and confident parent.

And guess what. The calmer and less stressed you are, the more productive you will be. (Or, if it seems more compelling to you this way: the higher the stress, the lower the productivity.) Get more done to stay calmer; get calmer to get more done.

There's no magic formula for managing your time. The basic idea is to take note of all the things you do, or need to do, and schedule them. Set them in your agenda as important appointments, just as you would do for work. Designate a time and a length of time for each thing. And *do not* cancel! When it feels like there's not enough time, this is how you make time.

CALENDARS

I have my calendar hung up on my office wall. For me, electronics just don't do it. I want to see everything all spread out. The visual helps me remember—and I find it motivating to see how many items I've accomplished and crossed out. Compare that to "tap and delete," which makes it like whatever thing you did was never there. And, it is harder to make excuses when I have to live with items that *aren't* crossed out posted up all month.

I admit the subtle pressure to complete the things I set out to do gives me the last little push I sometimes need to actually execute, rather than put off to another day.

You'll need a master calendar, for sure, and perhaps sub-calendars depending on what system you use, where and when you will need to refer to your calendar, whose activities you are tracking—and how it makes sense to your brain.

You will be noting in your chosen style of calendar (wall, electronic, desk, pocket, phone…) everything from daily happenings (school pickup) and regular activities (piano lesson) to once-in-a-while items (dental appointments and passport renewals). Be sure to include on the calendar anything you need to know about the appointment: address, contact info, what to bring with you…and you'll need not just your kids' stuff but yours too!

This is also the real secret to staying healthy when you are as busy as you are: schedule in time for all the things you do, or want to do, for healthy living—workout time, outdoor time, "me time," meal prep, family time, pajama days, vacations. Everything. Getting it on the calendar. Making an appointment with yourself increases the chances you will actually do it.

Here's another important thing about making time for everything this way: it proves to you there is time for it all. You will have to be thoughtful and realistic about what you give a time slot, how much time you allow, and where it is reasonable to fit it into your day. You probably have thirty minutes before bedtime, but are you really going to do that workout video then? Or, yes, you need to get to the grocery store, but is that really going to happen in the thirty minutes between the end of one soccer game and the beginning of another?

BE THERE

Whatever you need to do, take the time to do it right. Whatever task you're on, be in 100 percent.

JUST SAY NO

Here's another way to make more time out of not enough time: just say "no." Do it calmly and confidently. Because it's okay to say no to things. You do not have to do everything. Plan what you do, do what you plan, but don't add so many things to the calendar that you up your stress more than strictly necessary.

I try my best to be present wherever I am, whatever I am doing. When I am at work, I give it all my focus. When I'm at home with the kids, I keep my focus there. However frustrating it is for those trying to text me in the evening, my phone is usually put aside during those dinner and bedtime hours.

Stop multitasking! Doing two (or more) things at once can seem efficient and necessary, but it decreases the quality of what you are getting done. You create the illusion of getting a lot done while really accomplishing little, and you end up more, rather than less, stressed. It's no surprise to me that multitasking is one of the suspects on the list for what causes mom brain.

Focus on what needs to be done at the moment you are in. Focus on what's on your schedule for right now (not what's there for this time next week, or what was on there for yesterday).

SCHEDULING

Using a schedule, or following a routine, is another great way to keep chaos at bay. This should include all the items you are not going to put on your calendar, such as bedtime, when you have to be outside for the bus, when you leave for work, and "where am I going to fit in a shower?"

Is tooth brushing before or after story time? Is breakfast before or after getting dressed?

Once you have a schedule set up, follow it the best you can. You have to stay flexible because dinner is not always going to begin at six on the dot, no matter what schedule or routine you have in place. And that's okay. But having a regular routine sets everyone's expectations and eliminates a lot of day-to-day decision-making (and negotiation), which creates a calmer atmosphere for everyone. Which structure is best will vary from family to family and will shift over time.

I like putting my kids to bed a little later, for example, so I have that quality time in the evening after work and they sleep a little later into the morning. Since I like to take care of some things before they wake up for the day, this works for us. Other parents like their kids to go to sleep earlier so they have their evenings free and available for the same kind of stuff I'm dealing with in the mornings. The "right" way is the one that works best for your family.

SCHEDULE QUALITY TIME

When I am prioritizing, I always err on the side of creating quality time with my kids. What better way to focus your time management skills than toward time with family?

I calendar quality time like any other important commitment, and I protect it once it is in my schedule. I always aim to make the most of whatever time we do have together, even if it's not much. Any time we have together, I want to make it quality time.

To review: it is the quality of the time you have with your kids that counts. This is not a game measured in hours, days, or any unit of time. So, no mom guilt about exactly how much time you are with your kids.

SCHEDULE UNPLUGGED TIME

A great way to make more time in your day is to disconnect from your devices. In modern life, this is not something most of us can do all out or all of the time. You may have to monitor email for work or be available at all times by text for an aging parent. But, be honest, how much of your on-device time is time-wasting? And/or stressful? At the very least, you can't be on a device and be fully present to the moment you are in.

Far too many people are on screens even when they're

taking "me time," are on vacation, or are enjoying family time. Try making some time each day to disconnect, and you will reap the benefits of greater relaxation and productivity. And you'll have more time available to do what really matters to you—or at least to get stuff done.

LISTS, LISTS, AND MORE LISTS

If lists had a fan club, I'd be the president. Lists are a lifesaver for me. At certain points, I have lists of my lists, and I'm so into it I don't even care that sounds a bit ridiculous.

CUT THE CLUTTER

Think of all the times your children have had toys strewn around everywhere, though they had long ago moved on to play with something else. You're stepping over piles of throw pillows relocated from couch to floor to move backpacks from blocking the door. You feel frazzled, exhausted, and stressed.

The more mess is around, the more mess happens. The more mess happens, the more stress you feel.

Clutter not only takes up more time and energy when you are trying to find or clean things, but it also creates a feeling of chaos rather than calm. So clear it! Often it takes just a few minutes to put all the toys in one place, which immediately produces a sense of calm. In more serious cases of we-lost-control-of-the-clutter, you may have to declutter bit by bit, maybe one room at a time, or even section of room by section of room. Closet today, bookshelves tomorrow, before we even look to see what's under the bed... It'll be more than worth it.

Lists are how I create the kind of inside-your-brain organization I'm talking about. Just knowing I have everything written down and tracked, I'm calmer and more at ease, and I actually get more done. In fact, I don't think I'd ever get anything done without my lists, or I wouldn't even know where to start. My motto is, *Lists, or it doesn't happen.*

Lists create order, which leads to staying calm.

Lists make you more productive, helping you get things done rather than putting things off.

Lists give you organization and structure and a *plan* for your days, weeks, and long-term future.

Lists make you more likely to do items on it compared to when the list exists only in your head.

Lists help you prioritize, in order of importance, or timeliness, or both.

Lists help you see everything visually on your plate, in one quick view.

Lists help you set concrete goals.

Lists (or rather, checking things off lists) give you a sense of accomplishment, which, not for nothing, makes you more motivated to get other tasks done.

Lists can do so much in terms of the difference they make in your quality of life, which is the reason I'm telling you about my list dependence in this particular book. I don't know a more powerful way to infuse calm and confidence into mom life.

Lists reduce anxiety, a great feature in the midst of the chaos of mom life. Lists free up some space in your brain that might otherwise be devoted to maintaining a running tally of those floating tasks you *have* to get done. I have full confidence you can make much better use of that brain space!

If you haven't started making lists yet, now is a great time to put "Make Lists" in the top spot on your To Do list!

THE LIST OF LISTS

To avoid having a stressful and overwhelmingly long list that saps motivation and productivity, I suggest keeping a master list, a weekly list, and a daily list.

The master list should be all you need to do, regardless of when you need to get it done. I have had things hang out on my main list for months or even years! (Learn guitar, create family photo albums…) Go ahead and get down everything that is on your mind, for you, the kids, your home—whatever you need or want to take care of.

The weekly list is just that. What do you need to get done by the end of the week?

The daily list should be as simple as possible. This includes your must-dos for just today, whether that's finishing that project on deadline, calling your dad for his birthday, signing your kids up for after-school chess class, or buying milk. I put a note of the time I can get to each task, depending on the rest of my schedule that day.

You want to capture everything but also be able to see it all quickly. I prefer creating my daily list the night before. I swear it helps me sleep better.

I keep a notepad by my bed, too, so I can get down anything that comes to mind before bed. It's those thoughts running through our minds on a loop that keep us awake, and committing them to paper is usually enough to silence them at least enough to fall asleep.

There will always be new things to add to your list and things that need to move from one list to another. This is what I'm working on before I settle down for the night (*so* I can settle down for the night). But you'll also want to keep a list handy so you can add items whenever you think of them.

Keep a list on your phone or a kitchen whiteboard, send yourself voicemail, carry a little notebook—whatever works for you. I'm still a pen and paper list maker, but there is no one right medium. (If you use anything electronic, though, I strongly recommend getting one that is compatible with all devices you use.) Use what's comfortable and practical for you. The one thing I can tell you is not going to work is *I'll write that down later.*

WRITE IT DOWN

The simple act of writing a list will make it easier to remember to do things, even when you are not looking at your list. (Just in case I'm not the only one who goes to the store without the shopping list from time to time.) And the process of writing things down makes your memory's job easier. Research shows, for example, that if you are in a lecture or a conference and taking notes, you are more likely to remember it later on than if you were just listening to it. Your brain is taking in the information you are listening to, summarizing, and deciding which pieces of information to save for later. We remember information better by writing it down than if we were just listening to it or reading it.

Writing things down in an organized fashion brings even more benefits. It can help reduce stress because it relieves you of the fear you'll forget something. Research shows that simply making a plan to get things done—before actually doing anything about it—can free you from anxiety. When you write down what you need to do, you perform better and more effectively.

PRIORITIZE

Once you have your list system in place, you'll want to *prioritize* the items on the list in order of importance and timeliness.

Break down the things you need to do to make tasks more bite-sized, and keep goals realistic. "Plan Mom's 75th birthday party" isn't going to cut it. You need," create an invite email list," "order gift," "write a toast," and so forth. The more specific, the better. Just be sure to keep it realistic.

Don't carry an item on your daily to-do list if there's no chance you're going to get it done on that particular day. There's no, "get car inspection" on a day that's already jam-packed with kids' activities or appointments.

Indicate on your daily list the one or two things you absolutely *must* get done that day. I know the temptation is to start working through your list with what you know you can knock off the quickest, but that's not what I'm asking you to do here. What really *has* to be done on this particular day? (Go ahead and do some of the easy-peasy items, too—get that sense of accomplishment that comes from checking something off your list. It'll encourage you to keep going.)

For the day's true priorities, consider what matters to you. Recognize that what matters most to you may be different from day to day. Maybe you don't "*have*" to get to Zoom yoga class today because there's not a deadline involved or fines for not going. But if this is the day of the week your favorite instructor teaches, you can't really move this to another day without putting it off for a whole week. And you might really *need* yoga class—an hour devoted to that might put you right for the rest of the day. In that case, you might prioritize yoga over "renew driver's license." Even if there is only a week left until you are due to renew your license, you *can* deal with the DMV tomorrow, instead of today, if yoga means that much to you.

Once a task is on your daily or maybe even weekly list, it's time to make time for it. Just generally figure out a way you can make this happen. More specifically, mark a time for it on your calendar.

I recommend doing the top item or two on your daily list as early in the day as you possibly can. I offer the same reason I do for morning workouts: whatever you do early in the day is taken care of the rest of the day. That way, whichever way your day goes off the rails (because, when doesn't it?), you'll have some stuff squared away already. The later you let something go, the easier it starts to be to procrastinate about it.

You will move entries from your master or weekly list as they increase in importance or near deadlines—or simply when you know you'll have time to get them done. It *will* all get done, eventually. Or, you will realize you don't need or want to do it anyway (create photo albums for each kid, who am I kidding??) and you can drop them off the list. I have had some items on my lists for years while I come to the realization that I'm not really going to do it or don't really need to do it.

Just don't expect to finish your list every day. I rarely do! There are still only twenty-four hours in a day, and many of them are not going to unfold with perfect efficiency. In fact, some days, exactly nothing is going to get done, and that's just the way it is.

Life is full and can change quickly. If you get two things done off your list, great! You got your kid to the dentist, reviewed that document that's been awaiting your signature—hurray! If "email mom tribe for new accountant recommendations" didn't happen today, oh well. Tomorrow is another day.

These lists serve as organizers and backup memory, so they are valuable whether or not you complete them. Knowing you've captured all you need to get done can make what you have to get done feel less overwhelming, even before you have worked your way through even the first item.

With a structure in place to strive for and fall back on, you can expect the unexpected and flex as things shift, while hardly even breaking a sweat.

8

CALM AND CONFIDENT PARENTING IN A CRISIS

Picture my little guy, a preschooler, sick, sick, sick with flu and a throat so sore he had no voice left to even call out for me. His fever was up and down all night, with "down" hovering around 104 degrees. I was full on in Dr. Mom mode, alternating acetaminophen and ibuprofen, refreshing the cool (*not* cold) compress, repeatedly checking his temperature, lying on the floor next to his bed when he was able to fall asleep for a while and I, of course, remained wide awake, despite my exhaustion.

I still remember so clearly looking at the thermometer and seeing it register 105.8. It took my breath for a minute.

I knew he was burning up, but whoa! It was the highest temp he'd ever run.

Even given the general chaos known as mom life, sometimes things are really and truly going off the rails. When a day veers into an actual crisis, your calm and confident parenting skills are put to the test. Your goal is finding that "calm and confident" zone even if you're cleaning up vomit (again!) or tracking down a kid whose bus is really late or experiencing your own tough times.

Not that you sail serenely through emergencies, but that you are able to take care of business, do what you need to do, and be there with your child in ways that best support them, despite difficult circumstances and without projecting your own emotions in ways that increase their distress.

Staying (and looking and sounding) absolutely calm and confident may not always be possible. In those situations, the goal is to find your way back to that zone as you can. Accessing calm and confidence even in extremes will always help. But when you can't get all the way there, keep in mind that losing it will only make things worse. Sometimes, "keep it together" is as good as you can do—and that will be good enough.

I've had my share of alarming moments with my kids, with

that 105.8 thermometer reading one of the top ten. It is so scary seeing your kid so sick! Even with my professional knowledge, I feel anxiety and stress. And with emotions running high in those moments, it is harder than ever for parents to know exactly what to do. *Do I need to call the doctor? Do I need to go to the emergency room? How can I comfort my child?*

That fever felt like a crisis to me, and I *did* know (technically speaking) exactly what to do. It was yet another reminder for me about how tough such situations are on all parents. How does anyone ever manage these things? Especially when they happen so often in the middle of the night, so you're sleep deprived as well as uncertain and on the verge of panic.

It is normal to feel stressed and nervous when you are at crisis points, when your kid is sick or injured or the family is otherwise in some kind of distress. Of *course* you are going to feel stressed. Feeling that stress is not, by itself, a problem. In fact, this is the good type of stress—the kind that motivates you to get your butt in gear to solve the problem. Still, you want to be able to respond to a crisis as productively as you can.

I've learned a handful of strategies that have seen me through some of the most urgent dilemmas of our family life. They are:

DR. GOOGLE

Here's an anti-recommendation for staying calm in a crisis: *don't* rely on "Dr. Google" to diagnose or treat your kids (or yourself). Sure, internet sources can be useful for educating yourself about the care they, or you, are receiving, or connecting to others dealing with similar situations, for moral support. But when substituted for direct advice from health care professionals, there's a high likelihood of internet "advice" amping up anxiety, rather than assuaging it.

One common scenario: unnecessary worry created by looking up common signs, symptoms, or test results and finding a raft of possible diagnoses, including alarming ones. Worse still, trying to diagnose and treat yourself can be dangerous and detrimental to your health if you don't have the correct information, context, and judgment. Additionally, it is not always easy to gauge the accuracy, reliability, and trustworthiness of internet sources. Best to consult a professional before jumping to conclusions or choosing a course of action.

Acknowledge stress points. It's okay to admit you are stressed or that life is imperfect in some way (or ways!). What's true is true. Trying to paper over an issue or pretend it doesn't exist is often the source of the biggest part of the stress, even more than the thing itself. It's the mom version of "the cover-up is worse than the crime."

Have a plan. And a backup plan, and a plan to back up your backup plan. The sitter calls in sick—how's that for a mom emergency? If you know in advance what you are going to do—a "plan B" (and C and D)—then when the issue comes up, you can handle it with a minimum of fuss:

just phone a friend, draft a grandparent, ask your assistant to rearrange your calendar for a work-from-home day... whatever it is.

When I became a single mom, one of the worries that plagued me was: What if I have to take one kid to the ER someday? What am I going to do with the other kid? How could I take care of both while one was in crisis? I couldn't rest easy about this scenario until I made backup plans and put the relevant numbers in my phone in an "emergency contacts" section. And these are plans I have already put into action on at least one occasion.

Line up outside support. The time my son capped off a play date by falling and hitting his face on the monkey bars, requiring stitches, a friend stepped in to take my daughter to her house while my son and I went to the ER. Just as she'd said she would when I talked to her about it while it was still a hypothetical situation in which I might need her help one day. Let's hear it for the mom tribe!

Outside help of all kinds is important to set up. That's true for many reasons (moral support, handling normal logistics and time management, solving non-urgent problems that require expertise...) but high among them is allowing you to handle a crisis with relative calm: you have help on hand and others who will know what to do even if you are not sure. Your team may include sitters, friends, relatives who don't live with you, consultants, doctors, therapists, neighbors…the list goes on, and you will know better than anyone else who would be helpful when you need that extra hand.

Fake it 'til you make it. So, okay, even if you are *not* calm, you are going to want to *look* calm. You are going to speak calmly. You are going to act calmly. And eventually everyone, including you, will settle down.

Ask for help. The above points only work when you are willing to ask for help. Find the support you need, and then call on it as necessary. Choose your sources carefully, but then trust them. You do not have to do this parenting thing alone. In fact, it is next to impossible to do it alone. Trying to do it alone is likely to undermine calm and confidence, just when you need it most.

Have essentials on hand. If you can quickly grab whatever you need to deal with an emergency, you're that much more likely to be able to proceed with calm and confidence. Compare that to frantically searching for a thermometer or the records of your child's last weigh-in so you know the right dose of medicine—not calm- or confidence-friendly! Set yourself up with a good first aid kit, for example, and designate the specific place it definitely, permanently lives.

**Learn what calms *you* and your child when the chips are

down. Take a breath. Take a minute to yourself if you can. Take the first steps toward a solution. And here's a simple thing to try: lower the volume. Whatever you are saying, say it in a regular tone. Similar to "fake it 'til you make it," sounding as if you are calm (even if you are not) can actually calm you, as well as those around you. Bonus: when you speak calmly, everyone will hear you better.

EMERGENCY PHONE LIST

Compile a list of key contact information to reach:

- Each parent
- Pediatrician
- Any other doctors who follow your children
- Poison control
- Local ER/hospital
- Close family and/or trusted friends (identify who and where they are, in case someone other than you is making use of this list)

Your phone will also have these numbers, of course—or should if it doesn't already—but just in case it is out of sight, or charge, and in case someone other than you needs this info, a few hard copies of this list are important to have around.

Keep one with each first aid kit (see "In Case of Emergency"), and post in a central place or places in your home (including near your landline phone, if you have one). Anyone who ever cares for your children, formally or informally—grandparents, friends, and regular sitters—should also have a copy of this list. You should keep extras on hand to give anyone new, like a sitter or a neighbor watching your child for the first time.

Don't forget to update the list (and all copies of the list) as necessary.

Be aware of your child's emotions in a crisis—and your influence on them in those moments. I heard from a mom whose kid had a trip to the ER after an incident on the school playground. When the school called the mom to alert her, she absolutely wigged out at the school about their handling of the situation. She was scared and upset, so I could see how it happened, but the mom regretted her outburst. Her kid had gotten increasingly upset seeing how upset her mom was. As the mom reeled herself in, she was better able to be there for her child and do all the things she had to do to get the right care for her daughter as quickly as possible.

A BIG MESS

What counts as not just everyday chaos but an actual crisis will vary a bit from person to person and family to family—different things stress different people out in different ways. No matter where your threshold is, you are going to face crises both large and small that require urgent action. And of course, not all of them are medical.

Like the time my kids and I finally got around to changing the water in the fish tank.

We were delinquent in this chore, so the water was at the maximum grossness still compatible with life (for the fish). Also, we had just gotten a new living room rug at this point, so I bet you can see where this story is going.

IN CASE OF EMERGENCY

Knowing you are prepared for basic emergencies—with a well-stocked first aid kit and common medications on hand, so you'll be able to respond on short notice—will help you stay calmer during an urgent situation. What exactly to include may shift depending on the age of your child. And, as always, consult with your pediatrician about any medications, including over-the-counter.

- Acetaminophen and ibuprofen
- Syringe-type dispenser for giving medication
- Sunblock (over six months of age)
- Calamine and/or hydrocortisone cream for bug bites
- Benadryl or antihistamine
- Pedialyte oral rehydration (liquid or ice pops are great to have stocked in the fridge and freezer at home)

Keep a few complete first aid kits—one at home, one in the car, and one in the diaper bag, for example. Buying a pre-made first aid kit is one good way to get the key basics all in one go, and you can simply add to it whatever else you need or want. Following is a list of what to make sure is in your kit:

- Basic first aid manual (make sure it is up to date)
- Thermometer
- Vaseline or petroleum jelly
- Nail file or nail clippers (my preference is for a nail file)
- Alcohol wipes (to clean the thermometer and other tools)
- Brush or comb
- Sterile gauze pads
- Adhesive tape and small scissors
- Alcohol wipes
- Band-Aids in a variety of sizes and shapes
- Flashlight (cell phones can work too)
- Disposable ice pack
- Tweezers and/or safety pins
- Diaper cream
- Baby wipes
- Antibiotic ointment

We dropped the fish tank.

My grip slipped, on the hardwood floor right next to the new rug, and shards of glass and filthy water seemed to cover the whole room. The fish was flopping around on the floor, and I did not think it was going to survive.

This was not a life-and-death emergency—except, of course, for the fish. This was of grave concern to my children. They were upset, and I felt pretty panicked too. Urgent action was required.

I grabbed the first bowl I could reach in our kitchen, ran in some tap water, and scooped the fish into it. Once the fish was restored to water, the kids seemed better right away. It looked like the fish would make it. I, however, was worried about all that sharp glass and the sheer mess—it still felt like a bit of an emergency to me! Could we save the new rug? How long would we be haunted by the tiniest pieces of glass? Would our home ever not smell like fish poop? Would my children ever again attempt this chore?

I wasn't going to call in outside help for this, and I admit "fish poop on the rug" was not one of the situations I had made backup plans about, not even with shattered glass thrown in. I did have relevant essentials on hand—my daughter was a puker when she was really small, so I have long kept a corner of a closet devoted to stuff-for-getting-grossness-out-of-textiles. Taking the one concrete action to improve things (getting out cleaning supplies) was in itself a bit calming. I knew what to do. I was prepared to do it. It was going to work, and there was an endpoint in sight. Getting things as much under my control as I can is one of the strategies I know calms me.

I also acknowledged my distress, as calmly as I could, to my children. I may have been decidedly uncalm while the fish was out of water, so I owned that and talked through my reaction briefly:

"Wow, I was so scared for Nemo there. I felt bad for dropping him and worried I didn't know how to fix the situation. And a little afraid to touch him! I'm so relieved to see Nemo swimming around again. But, oh boy, what a mess this is, what a pain to have to clean it up! I'm glad we have the cleaning supplies here and that at least we can work together. But first stay over there while I deal with the glass…"

I didn't want to hide—couldn't hide—my stress, but I also didn't want to further stress my children. Talking through my feelings with them had a bonus to it: a model for them about how they might process their emotions, in those moments, but also in life generally. A thousand lessons like that, over time, is how they develop their ability to regulate themselves.

It wasn't long before we added one last strategy to the situation: we found the humor in it.

Once the fish was saved, the glass swept up, and the cleanup underway, we could look for the light spots of the situation. Turns out, making funny faces to reenact the fish's reaction to taking flight was pure comedy gold to us that day. There's no better way to defuse tension than to laugh it out. Not appropriate to every emergency, but when it's available, I highly recommend it.

TANTRUMS

A mom I know was pretty thrown the day her daughter Laila threw a huge tantrum when presented with the incorrect after-school snack. How was she supposed to handle that kind of intensity over that kind of ordinary occurrence? Laila, though, learned an important lesson that day about throwing a tantrum: it worked. The sugary snack was given as a peace offering, teeing up a repeat the next day. Prostrate on the floor, top volume moaning and crying, the works.

The only one more miserable than Laila appeared to be was her mother, who, about two minutes in, felt like this would never end. How was she supposed to stay calm in the middle of this?

Tantrums themselves are not a big danger to your child

or to you. But, especially when they occur in public, they can certainly *feel* like an emergency! Not only is everyone watching, and, you imagine, judging your parenting, but also you may fear the out-of-control movements that can come along with them might pose injury risk. You may risk being whacked by a flailing body part, or you may worry your kid is going to crack their head open the way they are flinging themselves around the floor.

Tantrums can take a toll on everyone, and on the level of calm and confidence in the household. For a parent, a tantrum can feel like an overwhelming, exhausting eternity. Once they are set off, there isn't much you can do to stop the speeding train of a tantrum. The same goes for the not-technically-tantrums bad-behavior storms you see in older kids.

But it will stop. (And kids tend to bounce right back after, even if their parents still feel frazzled hours later).

Practicing calm and confident parenting does not mean your child will never again have a tantrum. And it doesn't mean you won't be stressed by a tantrum. It means that while your child is having a tantrum, you can be calm and confident in how you are responding to it. It means you can acknowledge that it's stressful without denying the problem or melting down yourself. It means you can think about how to take care of yourself through the situation, as well as your kid. It's the usual foundational principle of calm and confident parenting: you care for yourself so that you can do your best in caring for your child. Even when things get really rough.

The calm and confident approach to a tantrum is straightforward: don't engage. Once a tantrum starts, there's not much you can really do; they won't hear you until they are calmer. As long as they are not, in fact, hurting themselves or others, ignore them the best you can. Let your kid whine, cry, scream, or whatever else they are doing to release the stress they are dealing with. Stay calm the best you can. Try not to be reactive.

Don't pressure yourself not to feel stressed by a tantrum; that's not the goal, because it is a stressful situation. But keep your cool anyway. Because if you act all stressed out, that's going to make it all worse. The whole tantrum will go on longer, or intensify, or recur sooner or more often.

The calm and confident parent, faced with a tantrum, does not stress about how they are doing as a parent, or the way they are handling the immediate circumstances, or life in general. They do not worry if they are doing what they are "supposed" to do. They do not worry about whatever any witnesses are making of the situation. They definitely don't try to create a "teaching moment" during a tantrum. (That comes later after the child is calm again and will be able to actually hear and process and remember what you are saying, which they simply cannot do while worked up.)

The calmer you can remain, the better your child will be able to calm themselves.

KEEP YOUR COOL

The night my son was so sick, I felt my own heart race when I saw the thermometer readout at 105.8. I forced myself to take a breath then review medical facts so I could choose my course of action calmly. Or, at least calmly enough to appear calm to my son, for however much he was paying attention. And within a few hours, the fever went down and stayed down, and he was soon on the mend.

Whether it's illness or injury, a sitter no-show, an endangered pet, a public meltdown, or a temperature rising, you can keep your cool even when things are otherwise going wrong. The ways of the calm and confident parent will carry you through crisis as well as the more typical kinds of everyday chaos.

CONCLUSION

You aren't supposed to know how to parent. You aren't born knowing how to do it, you don't really get taught it, and no one makes you get licensed or insured before handing over a kid to you. So yes, there's a lot to learn, you won't always know exactly what you are doing, and it's often overwhelming, while also totally amazing.

This kid is my responsibility…what if I mess this up?

The reality is, there isn't a way to do this correctly. There's no user manual, no guarantee, no bible. You can get all kinds of information and advice, you can find lots of great models around you, but at some level, *you are making this up.*

Every mom has to find what works and doesn't work for her,

her child, and her family. When you bring your best self to this game, you get the best results for everyone. That's why I ground my message for moms in the idea that taking care of themselves is the first and best way to take care of their families. And why I want to share the information parents need to parent calmly and with full confidence.

When I was way pregnant with my second child, I had an injury that had my foot in a boot for weeks on end. There I was, big-bellied, limping, pushing a budding toddler around the streets of Manhattan in a stroller…and getting literally stopped on the street and asked how in the world I was still smiling. I'm not totally sure I even know, since many of those days I spent thinking about how much I wanted to go workout, or sleep.

Somewhere in there, pushed into it by a series of unfortunate events I wouldn't wish on anybody, I figured out how to stay calm in the midst of the chaos. I'm someone who really likes feeling in control, but I learned fast after becoming a parent that there was a lot I just wasn't in charge of. Fighting that fact didn't help. Moving through it calmly, or at least *aiming* for calm, did.

This realization was a game-changer for me as a mom, and the pediatrician in me wanted to help other families find this same lane. If there's a more important single component to a kid growing up all-around healthy, I don't know what it is.

But it is not always easy to access. Every time I feel out of my depth in some parenting decision, situation, mishap, or crisis, I'm reminded that, compared to a lot of parents, I've got more resources on board thanks to my medical background. Sometimes it's still a challenge for me to find calm and confidence, even knowing which is the right medication, or what the experts say about how to respond to a child who just told you they are being teased by classmates. How in the world are other parents supposed to manage, much less stay calm about it?

I'm on a mission to help. I want other parents to know it's possible to find calm and confidence, even when life is in chaos.

Is it hard? It can be. But absolutely worth it. When patients, friends, and family have called me with panicked questions about their kids, the feedback I always get is how much relief it brought them to talk it over. And how much better they feel overall when they experience that calm in the wake of panic.

It's not so much the information I gave them, even though it was needed. I think what parents react to most is my calmness. It always stood out to me how much the ability to find that calm meant to parents.

I want to give you the tools to parent calmly and confidently by balancing caring for yourself and caring for your children. I want you to make the changes that, small as they may be, will make big impacts on your life and your family life. I want you to let go of your fear that you're somehow screwing this up.

I spent a long time in the wake of my series of personal health crises stuck in, "Why is this happening to me?" But I've learned a lot through the process, sometimes in surprising but life-changing ways, and I've ended up somewhere around, "Everything happens for a reason."

As hard as it got at points, it changed who I was as a person and a parent—and all for the better. I would never have been the parent I am today had I not gone through all of what I've gone through. I would be parenting very differently, and I think my kids wouldn't be the same, either. I definitely would not be able to be as calm as I (usually) find a way to be now, through clothing-related tantrums, cracker-crumb snowstorms, skyrocketing fevers, missed buses, burnt dinners, and the like.

So take care of yourself first. Eat right, move your body regularly, get some sleep, and get organized. Find time for it. *Make* time for it. Get the benefits for yourself, and see how they flow down to your kids.

Let doing right by yourself give you the confidence that you are a good parent, making good decisions, and sometimes just rolling with it—because what else are you going to do? Some days calm will be an illusion or an aspiration, but the quest for it should always move you in the right direction.

Then, when you look back on the day, or year, or entire childhood, it will be with awe and gratitude for how much you love these little people and how lucky and thankful you feel to be their mom. And even on the days when there's been a struggle or uncertainty, in the rearview, you'll find you loved every minute of it all.

This is the best part of calm and confident parenting: that it allows you to fully engage with and enjoy mom life.

Chaos and all.

ACKNOWLEDGMENTS

I would like to thank everyone who has been a part of making this book happen and helped along the way.

My family and friends and mom tribe and sitters, who were all so supportive.

Julie, for always being an eye and ear for feedback when I needed it.

My children, for their excitement about this book and always keeping me accountable and making sure I kept to my timeline.

Caren, for being the best friend all these years, our endless chats, and being a part of every step of the way.

Hillary, Hope, and Debbie, for always being there for me and my kids anytime anywhere.

Dad and Linda, for the listening and advice.

Everyone on the Scribe team who has helped me so much. Special thanks to Tucker, Hal, Colleen, Emily, and Natalie.

My mentors, for inspiring me to get to where I am today.

To all of those I have had the opportunity to lead, teach, and mentor over my career and have been the inspiration and motivation for this book.

It is impossible to list everyone. Know that I am truly grateful for you all.

ABOUT THE AUTHOR

DR. ALISON MITZNER is a single mom, pediatrician, family wellness and fitness expert, and passionate supporter of moms feeling calm, confident, and healthy. She has worked with over 6,000 patients and reaches millions of people with her fitness, health, and wellness information for moms of all types—new, single, stay-at-home, working, and just plain busy.

Dr. Mitzner has been featured in *Forbes*, *The Huffington Post*, *Reader's Digest*, *Shape*, *Parents*, *Self*, *Today*, Fox News, CNN, MSN, What to Expect, Romper, The Everymom, Aaptiv, and more.

After attending medical school in Syracuse and completing her residency on Long Island, Dr. Mitzner worked at a busy private practice in Manhattan, New York. She is currently a senior director at a major pharmaceutical company. Outside of supporting parents, she loves being a mom, spending time with her two kids, singing, and staying active, including dancing, playing sports, and really any fitness activity.

Visit Dr. Alison Mitzner on the web:
www.dralisonmitzner.com

Connect with Dr. Alison Mitzner on social media:
@dralisonmitzner

www.ingramcontent.com/pod-product-compliance
Lightning Source LLC
Chambersburg PA
CBHW060526080526
44586CB00012B/633